SEROTONIN-BOOSTING FOODS & COOKBOOK

DELICIOUS RECIPES FOR A JOYFUL MIND

HELEN E. JACQUES

CONTENTS:

INTRODUCTION

Serotonin, often referred to as the "feel-good" neurotransmitter, plays a crucial role in regulating mood, appetite, and sleep. As a medical professional, I am well aware of the impact serotonin levels can have on overall well-being. In this article, I will provide a comprehensive overview of serotonin-boosting foods, drawing from both professional medical knowledge and my personal experience. Understanding how certain foods can positively influence serotonin production can help us make informed dietary choices for improved mental health.

Serotonin is synthesized from the amino acid tryptophan, which is obtained through dietary sources. Consuming foods rich in tryptophan can provide the necessary building blocks for serotonin production in the brain. Additionally, these foods work in synergy with other nutrients and factors to optimize serotonin synthesis.

Here are some serotonin-boosting foods that you can incorporate into your diet:

Complex Carbohydrates: Foods such as whole grains, legumes, and starchy vegetables like sweet potatoes contain high levels of complex carbohydrates. These foods stimulate the release of insulin, which promotes the uptake of most amino acids in the body, except for tryptophan. Consequently, this increases the availability of tryptophan in the brain and enhances serotonin production.

Protein-Rich Foods: Protein sources like lean poultry, fish, eggs, and dairy products contain tryptophan, which serves as a precursor for serotonin. Combining these protein-rich foods with carbohydrates can further enhance tryptophan absorption and utilization.

Nuts and Seeds: Walnuts, almonds, flaxseeds, and chia seeds are excellent sources of tryptophan. Additionally, they provide essential omega-3 fatty acids, which are important for overall brain health and serotonin function.

Fruits and Vegetables: Bananas, pineapples, kiwis, and tomatoes are known to contain vitamins and minerals that support serotonin production. These fruits and vegetables are rich in vitamin C, which aids in the conversion of tryptophan to serotonin.

Dark Chocolate: Dark chocolate, particularly in varieties with high cocoa content, is not only a delicious treat but also a natural mood booster. It contains tryptophan and other compounds that can stimulate serotonin production and release in the brain.

As a medical professional, I have witnessed the positive impact of serotonin-boosting foods on my patients' mental health. Moreover, I have personally incorporated these foods into my diet and experienced their benefits. By regularly consuming a balanced diet that includes the aforementioned serotonin-boosting foods, I have noticed improvements in my overall mood, energy levels, and sleep quality. I find that incorporating these foods into my meals and snacks allows me to maintain a stable and positive outlook, even during stressful periods.

It is important to note that while serotonin-boosting foods can contribute to improved mental well-being, they should not replace professional medical care or therapy when necessary. For individuals with severe serotonin imbalances or mental health disorders, it is crucial to consult with a healthcare professional for appropriate diagnosis and treatment.

Serotonin-boosting foods can be a valuable addition to a healthy and balanced diet. Incorporating complex carbohydrates, protein-rich foods, nuts and seeds, fruits and vegetables, and dark chocolate into your meals can support serotonin production and promote a positive mood. However, it is essential to approach mental health holistically, seeking professional guidance when needed. By combining the benefits of serotonin-boosting foods with comprehensive medical care, we can take proactive steps toward enhancing our overall well-being.

SEROTONIN AND HOW IT AFFECT MOOD

A neurotransmitter called serotonin is essential for controlling several physiological processes in the body, such as mood, appetite, sleep, and cognition. Its impact on mood and emotional health has earned it the nickname "feel-good" neurotransmitter. We will delve into the specifics of serotonin and how it influences mood in this extensive article.

Tryptophan, an amino acid that can be found in foods, is converted into serotonin in the body. Once tryptophan reaches the brain, it goes through a series of chemical processes to become serotonin. Enzymes, vitamins, and cofactors aid in this conversion process. The production of serotonin can be significantly influenced by the availability of tryptophan and the activity of these enzymes.

Serotonin functions as a modulator in the brain, affecting the activity of other neurotransmitters and regulating mood. It contributes to the regulation of neurotransmitter levels, including those of dopamine and norepinephrine, which are linked to motivation, pleasure, and alertness. Serotonin promotes happiness, contentment, and emotional stability when levels are at their highest.

Serotonin deficiencies have been linked to several mood disorders, including anxiety and depression. Serotonin dysregulation is thought to play a role in the emergence of these conditions, despite thought exact causes are complex and multifactorial. Serotonin levels are frequently found to be below average in depressed people. Symptoms such as protracted sadness, a loss of interest in activities, exhaustion, and adjustments to appetite and sleep patterns may result from this.

The success of some medications in treating depression and anxiety is additional evidence that serotonin influences mood. Antidepressant medications in the selective serotonin reuptake inhibitor (SSRI) class work by making more serotonin available in the brain. These drugs prevent serotonin from being reabsorbed, allowing it to stay in the synaptic cleft between neurons for a longer period. In turn, this improves serotonin, signaling the mood of people with depressive disorders.

Serotonin affects appetite and satiety in addition to its function in mood regulation. Serotonin receptors are found in the hypothalamus, an area of the brain that controls satiety and hunger. Serotonin increases feelings of fullness and curbs appetite when it binds to these receptors. This is why some serotonin-boosting drugs, like some SSRIs, may temporarily alter appetite, resulting in fewer food cravings and possible weight loss.

Serotonin also plays a role in controlling sleep patterns. It promotes restful sleep and balances the sleep-wake cycle. Melatonin, a neurotransmitter well known for controlling sleep and wakefulness, is created when serotonin is converted into another neurotransmitter. As the sun sets, melatonin levels rise, alerting the body that it is time to sleep. This process can be hampered by low serotonin levels, which can cause insomnia.

Even though serotonin is crucial for mood regulation, it's important to realize that mood disorders are complicated conditions with many underlying causes. Dysregulation of serotonin is only a small part of a much bigger picture. Mood and mental health can also be influenced by other factors, such as genetic predisposition, environmental factors, stress, and lifestyle choices.

It is important to remember that serotonin and mood have a two-way relationship. Serotonin levels can also be influenced by our emotions and mood. Activities that increase happiness, social interaction, and self-care can have a positive effect on serotonin synthesis and release. Regular physical activity, exposure to sunlight, and taking part in interests or pursuits that bring happiness and fulfillment can all help serotonin function.

In conclusion, serotonin is an important neurotransmitter for controlling mood. Serotonin imbalances can contribute to mood disorders like depression and anxiety, while optimal levels are linked to feelings of well-being and emotional stability. Incorporating lifestyle choices, therapeutic interventions, and, when necessary, medical treatments into a holistic approach to mental health can help us better understand the complex relationship between serotonin and mood. This will support optimal serotonin function and general well-being.

HOW DIET IMPACT SEROTONIN LEVELS

Diet greatly affects how much serotonin is present in the body. The availability and production of serotonin can be affected by the consumption of particular nutrients, especially those necessary for its synthesis and metabolism. For mood and general mental health to be at their best, it is essential to comprehend how diet affects serotonin levels.

Availability of tryptophan: Tryptophan is a necessary amino acid and a building block of serotonin. Tryptophan can be made more available in the brain by eating foods high in it, which boosts serotonin production. Poultry, fish, dairy products, eggs, nuts, seeds, and legumes are among the foods high in tryptophan. Your diet can help serotonin synthesis if you consume these protein sources.

Insulin Release and Carbohydrate Intake: Indirect effects of carbohydrate intake on serotonin levels. Insulin is released when carbohydrates are consumed, and insulin facilitates the uptake of all amino acids into cells except tryptophan. The relative concentration of tryptophan rises in the bloodstream as other amino acids are absorbed, allowing for more tryptophan to enter the brain and be converted into serotonin. Whole grains, legumes, and starchy vegetables are excellent examples of complex carbohydrates that help increase the availability of tryptophan.

Micronutrients: Specific vitamins and minerals are necessary for the synthesis and operation of serotonin. For instance, vitamin B6 functions as a cofactor in the transformation of tryptophan into serotonin. Bananas, poultry, fish, spinach, and chickpeas are all excellent sources of vitamin B6. In addition, vitamin C, which is abundant in citrus fruits, berries, and bell peppers, is involved in the conversion of tryptophan to serotonin. For supporting serotonin production, it's critical to consume enough of these micronutrients.

Omega-3 Fatty Acids: It has been discovered that omega-3 fatty acids, in particular, eicosapentaenoic acid (EPA) and docosahexaenoic acid (DHA), support serotonin function and elevate mood. Walnuts, chia seeds, flaxseeds, and fatty fish (like salmon, mackerel, and sardines) are good sources of these good fats. Consuming these foods regularly can support healthy serotonin levels.

Gut-Brain Connection: Recent studies have suggested that gut microbiota may affect the availability and production of serotonin. The synthesis and metabolism of serotonin can be supported by a healthy gut microbiome. Consuming foods high in probiotics, such as yogurt, kefir, sauerkraut, and kimchi, can support gut flora and may have affect serotonin levels.

Hydration: It's crucial to maintain hydration for overall health, which includes having a healthy brain. The balance of neurotransmitters, including serotonin, can be impacted by dehydration. To support serotonin function, make sure you are drinking enough water throughout the day.

Although dietary changes can affect serotonin levels, it's important to remember that they might not be enough to treat severe mood disorders. Professional medical and psychological interventions are crucial in cases of clinical depression or anxiety. However, a comprehensive strategy for mental well-being can benefit from a balanced diet that includes nutrients that support serotonin.

To address specific dietary requirements and potential drug interactions, it is also essential to take individual variations into account and consult with a healthcare provider or registered dietitian. They can offer you individualized advice based on your particular situation and assist in developing a diet that promotes serotonin production and general mental health.

BENEFITS OF CONSUMING SEROTONIN-BOOSTING FOODS

Consuming serotonin-boosting foods offers several benefits for mental well-being and overall health. These foods provide the necessary nutrients and precursors for serotonin synthesis, supporting optimal serotonin levels in the brain.

Here are some key benefits of including serotonin-boosting foods in your diet:

Improved Mood: Serotonin is often referred to as the "feel-good" neurotransmitter due to its role in regulating mood. By consuming foods rich in tryptophan, such as lean proteins, nuts, and seeds, you can increase the availability of this essential amino acid in the brain. This, in turn, promotes serotonin production and can contribute to a more positive mood and emotional well-being.

Reduced Anxiety and Stress: Serotonin has a calming effect on the brain and can help reduce anxiety and stress levels. By incorporating serotonin-boosting foods into your diet, you can support a healthy balance of neurotransmitters and promote a sense of calm and relaxation. Foods such as complex carbohydrates (whole grains, legumes) and fruits and vegetables (bananas, pineapples, kiwis) can help in this regard.

Better Sleep Quality: Serotonin plays a crucial role in regulating sleep patterns. By consuming foods that support serotonin production, you can promote healthy sleep-wake cycles and improve sleep quality. Dark chocolate, for example, contains tryptophan and other compounds that can stimulate serotonin release and contribute to a more restful sleep.

Enhanced Cognitive Function: Serotonin is involved in cognitive processes such as memory, learning, and attention. Optimal serotonin levels can support cognitive function and promote mental clarity. By incorporating omega-3 fatty acid-rich foods (fatty fish, walnuts) into your diet, you can support serotonin function and potentially enhance cognitive abilities.

Increased Feelings of Well-being: Serotonin is closely linked to feelings of well-being and contentment. Consuming serotonin-boosting foods can contribute to a general sense of happiness and satisfaction. Including a variety of nutrient-dense foods in your diet, such as whole grains, lean proteins, fruits, vegetables, and nuts, can provide the necessary nutrients for serotonin synthesis and promote overall well-being.

Appetite Regulation: Serotonin plays a role in regulating appetite and satiety. By supporting serotonin production through dietary choices, you can potentially improve appetite control and reduce cravings. Protein-rich foods, such as poultry, fish, and dairy products, can provide tryptophan for serotonin synthesis while helping you feel fuller for longer.

Nutritional Benefits: Serotonin-boosting foods are often nutrient-dense and offer additional health benefits. For example, fruits and vegetables are rich in vitamins, minerals, and antioxidants, which support overall health and contribute to a well-balanced diet. Nuts and seeds provide essential fatty acids and other beneficial nutrients. By including these foods in your diet, you can reap the nutritional benefits along with the serotonin-boosting effects.

It is important to note that while consuming serotonin-boosting foods can support mental well-being, they should not replace professional medical care or therapy when necessary. For individuals with severe mood disorders or serotonin imbalances, it is crucial to seek appropriate diagnosis and treatment from healthcare professionals.

SEROTONIN BOOSTING FOODS

BANANAS

Due to their nutritional makeup and potential effect on serotonin production, bananas are frequently thought of as a food that raises serotonin levels. Neurotransmitter serotonin is essential for regulating mood, appetite, sleep, and general mental health. Let's examine in depth why and how bananas can support serotonin levels and why they are thought to be a food that increases serotonin:

Bananas are a good source of the essential amino acid tryptophan, which is needed for the synthesis of serotonin. Serotonin is produced in the brain from tryptophan, which helps control mood. Although bananas don't contain a lot of tryptophan compared to other foods, their presence in the fruit can still help the body make serotonin.

Vitamin B6: Pyridoxine, also known as vitamin B6, is present in bananas in significant amounts. A coenzyme known as vitamin B6 is involved in the synthesis of neurotransmitters like serotonin as well as other metabolic processes. A sufficient intake of vitamin B6 is required for the best serotonin synthesis. Bananas can assist in ensuring a sufficient intake of this crucial nutrient.

Bananas are a good source of dietary fiber, which may indirectly help serotonin levels. Blood sugar levels are better controlled and are less likely to fluctuate suddenly. It's crucial to keep blood sugar levels steady to encourage consistent serotonin production. By consuming bananas, you can promote stable blood sugar levels and perhaps even serotonin synthesis.

Bananas are frequently linked to a naturally uplifting effect on mood. Numerous factors may be responsible for this perception, even though the precise mechanisms are not fully understood. Bananas' tryptophan, vitamin B6, fiber content, and naturally sweet flavor may all work together to improve mood and general well-being.

Potassium: A vital mineral necessary for many physiological processes, including nerve and muscle function, bananas are a rich source of potassium. Since proper nerve function is essential for serotonin release and signaling, potassium may indirectly affect serotonin levels. Bananas can help maintain adequate potassium levels and may support serotonin balance when consumed as part of a balanced diet.

Other Nutrients: Bananas also contain potassium, fiber, vitamin B6, and tryptophan, among other vital vitamins and minerals. These include manganese, magnesium, and vitamin C, all of which are crucial for overall health and well-being. Even though they may not have as much of a direct effect on serotonin levels, a balanced diet is essential for optimum brain health and neurotransmitter production.

Bananas are a convenient choice for raising serotonin levels because they are a fruit that is both accessible and versatile. They can be used alone as a nutritious snack, as an ingredient in smoothies, in baking, or combination with other foods. They are an efficient option to include in a diet that supports serotonin because of their portability and long shelf life.

KEY NUTRIENTS IN BANANAS

Carbohydrates: Bananas are primarily composed of carbohydrates, making them an excellent source of energy. They contain both simple sugars (fructose, glucose, and sucrose) and complex carbohydrates, providing a steady release of energy.

Fiber: Bananas are a good source of dietary fiber. A medium-sized banana typically contains around 3 grams of fiber. Dietary fiber supports digestive health, helps regulate blood sugar levels, and promotes a feeling of fullness.

Potassium: Bananas are well-known for their potassium content. Potassium is an essential mineral that plays a crucial role in maintaining proper heart and muscle function, nerve transmission, and fluid balance. A medium-sized banana can provide approximately 400-450 mg of potassium.

Vitamin C: Bananas contain a moderate amount of vitamin C, an antioxidant that supports immune function, collagen synthesis, and iron absorption. A medium-sized banana usually provides around 10% of the recommended daily intake of vitamin C.

Vitamin B6: Bananas are a good source of vitamin B6, also known as pyridoxine. Vitamin B6 plays a vital role in various bodily functions, including the metabolism of proteins, carbohydrates, and neurotransmitters. It also supports brain development and function.

Magnesium: Bananas contain a small but notable amount of magnesium, an essential mineral involved in over 300 enzymatic reactions in the body. Magnesium is crucial for maintaining healthy bones, regulating blood pressure, and supporting muscle and nerve function.

Manganese: Bananas contain manganese, a trace mineral that acts as a cofactor for various enzymes involved in metabolism, antioxidant defense, and bone health.

Other Nutrients: Bananas also provide smaller amounts of other essential nutrients, including vitamin A, vitamin E, vitamin K, folate, niacin, riboflavin, and trace amounts of minerals like calcium, iron, zinc, and copper.

TRYPTOPHAN AND SEROTONIN SYNTHESIS:

1. Tryptophan is an essential amino acid found in bananas and acts as a precursor for serotonin production.
2. When consumed, tryptophan is converted into serotonin in the brain, contributing to mood regulation.
3. While bananas may not contain exceptionally high levels of tryptophan compared to other protein

sources, they still contribute to the overall pool of tryptophan available for serotonin synthesis.

VITAMIN B6 AND SEROTONIN PRODUCTION:

1. Bananas are a notable source of vitamin B6, also known as pyridoxine.
2. Vitamin B6 plays a crucial role as a coenzyme in the conversion of tryptophan into serotonin.
3. Adequate levels of vitamin B6 are essential for optimal serotonin production, and including bananas in the diet can help meet the body's vitamin B6 requirements.

FIBER CONTENT AND SEROTONIN REGULATION:

1. Bananas are a good source of dietary fiber, both soluble and insoluble.
2. Dietary fiber plays a role in regulating blood sugar levels, which can indirectly affect serotonin levels.
3. Stable blood sugar levels are important for maintaining steady serotonin production, and the fiber in bananas helps prevent rapid spikes and drops in blood sugar.

HEALTH BENEFITS OF BANANA

Bananas have a rich nutritional profile, which makes them beneficial for your health in many ways. Including bananas in your diet can promote general health and support several different aspects of well-being following are some of the main health advantages of eating bananas:

Rich in nutrients: Bananas are a great source of dietary fiber, vitamins, and minerals. They are a fantastic source of magnesium, potassium, vitamin C, and vitamin B6. These nutrients are essential for supporting a variety of bodily processes and advancing general health.

Heart Health: Bananas are good for your heart because they are high in potassium. Having healthy blood pressure is important for lowering the risk of cardiovascular diseases like hypertension and stroke. Potassium helps maintain these levels. Bananas' high fiber content also promotes cardiovascular health by lowering cholesterol levels and enhancing all cardiovascular functions.

Digestive Health: Bananas are renowned for having a high fiber content, which helps to keep the digestive system in good shape. Bananas' soluble and insoluble fiber encourages normal bowel movements and guards against constipation. Pectin, a naturally occurring substance found in bananas, serves as a prebiotic by promoting the development of good gut bacteria.

Energy Boost: Natural sugars like glucose, fructose, and sucrose found in bananas give you a quick and long-lasting energy boost. Athletes frequently use them as a natural energy source to improve their performance and endurance while working out.

Mood Enhancement: Tryptophan and vitamin B6 are two nutrients found in bananas that have been shown to have mood-enhancing properties. An amino acid called tryptophan is converted by the body into serotonin, a neurotransmitter that affects mood regulation and feelings of well-being. Serotonin is one of the neurotransmitters whose synthesis is aided by vitamin B6.

Weight management: Because they are high in fiber, bananas can help with weight management. By encouraging feelings of fullness and satiety, the fiber lowers the risk of overeating and unhealthy snacking. Additionally, compared to processed snacks and desserts, bananas are naturally sweet and filling.

Improved Exercise Performance: Bananas are a great pre- and post-workout snack due to the natural sugars, electrolytes, and nutrients they contain. While potassium and magnesium help maintain proper muscle function and avoid muscle cramps, the hydrates offer easily accessible energy.

Eye Health: Bananas are rich in antioxidants like vitamins A and C which are good for the eyes. These vitamins and minerals support clear vision and overall eye health by helping to shield the eyes from oxidative stress and age-related macular degeneration.

Bone Health: Bananas contain several minerals, such as manganese and magnesium, which are crucial for maintaining strong bones. These minerals support bone strength and density, which lowers the risk of diseases like osteoporosis.

Blood Sugar Control: Bananas contain natural sugars, but their fiber content helps delay the blood sugar's absorption into the body. This may improve blood sugar regulation and lessen the likelihood of unexpected blood sugar spikes.

Although bananas have many health advantages, it's important to remember that everyone has different nutritional needs. To ensure adequate nutrient intake, it is crucial to include bananas in a balanced diet that also includes a variety of other fruits, vegetables, whole grains, lean proteins, and healthy fats.

Nuts and Seeds

Nuts and seeds are considered excellent serotonin-boosting foods due to their nutrient-rich profiles and ability to provide key precursors for serotonin synthesis. Including a variety of nuts and seeds in your diet can have several benefits for mood regulation and overall mental well-being. Let's delve into why nuts and seeds are regarded as serotonin-boosting foods:

TRYPTOPHAN CONTENT:

- Nuts and seeds, such as almonds, walnuts, sunflower seeds, and pumpkin seeds, are rich sources of tryptophan.
- Tryptophan is an essential amino acid that serves as a precursor for serotonin production in the brain.
- By consuming nuts and seeds, you can increase your intake of tryptophan and support serotonin synthesis.

HEALTHY FATS:

- Nuts and seeds are abundant in healthy fats, including omega-3 fatty acids and monounsaturated fats.
- Omega-3 fatty acids, found in walnuts, flaxseeds, and chia seeds, are beneficial for brain health and can support serotonin function.
- Monounsaturated fats, present in almonds and cashews, help maintain a healthy balance of neurotransmitters, including serotonin.

NUTRIENT DENSITY:

- Nuts and seeds are packed with essential nutrients, such as vitamins, minerals, and antioxidants.
- B vitamins, including vitamin B6 and folate, are particularly important for serotonin synthesis, and many nuts and seeds contain these nutrients.
- Additionally, minerals like magnesium and zinc, found in cashews, almonds, and pumpkin seeds, play a role in supporting serotonin production.

FIBER CONTENT:

- Nuts and seeds are excellent sources of dietary fiber, which aids in digestion and helps regulate blood sugar levels.
- Stable blood sugar levels are essential for optimal serotonin production and mood regulation.
- Consuming nuts and seeds can contribute to steady energy levels and prevent blood sugar fluctuations that may negatively affect serotonin balance.

VERSATILITY AND VARIETY:

- Nuts and seeds offer a wide range of options, allowing for versatility in incorporating them into your diet.
- They can be enjoyed as snacks on their own, added to salads, yogurts, or smoothies, or used as ingredients in baking and cooking.
- Adding a variety of nuts and seeds to your meals and snacks ensures a diverse nutrient intake, supporting overall health and well-being.

PORTABILITY AND CONVENIENCE:

- Nuts and seeds are portable and convenient, making them an easy and accessible serotonin-boosting snack option.
- They can be carried with you wherever you go, providing a nutritious and satisfying snack on the go.

BALANCED DIET AND INDIVIDUAL CONSIDERATIONS:

- While nuts and seeds offer numerous benefits, it is important to incorporate them as part of a balanced diet that includes a variety of serotonin-boosting foods.
- Individual responses to serotonin-boosting foods may vary, and it is crucial to consider personal dietary needs and preferences.

HEALTH BENEFITS OF NUTS AND SEEDS

Nuts and seeds have been linked to several health benefits, including:

Reduced risk of heart disease: Nuts and seeds are a good source of healthy fats, which can help lower cholesterol levels and reduce the risk of heart disease.

Reduced risk of type 2 diabetes: Nuts and seeds can help improve blood sugar control, which may help reduce the risk of type 2 diabetes.

Reduced risk of obesity: Nuts and seeds can help you feel full and satisfied, which may help you lose weight or maintain a healthy weight.

Reduced risk of certain types of cancer: Nuts and seeds may help reduce the risk of certain types of cancer, such as breast cancer and prostate cancer.

Improved brain health: Nuts and seeds may help improve brain function and memory.

Improved skin health: Nuts and seeds may help improve skin health by reducing inflammation and protecting the skin from damage from the sun.

DARK CHOCOLATE

Dark chocolate is not only a delectable treat but also a surprising source of potential mood-boosting benefits. With its rich, indulgent flavor and velvety texture, dark chocolate has captivated taste buds around the world. Beyond its irresistible taste, dark chocolate contains compounds that may positively affect our mood and overall well-being. We will explore the fascinating relationship between dark chocolate and mood enhancement, shedding light on the science behind its potential benefits.

THE SCIENCE OF DARK CHOCOLATE:

- Dark chocolate is derived from the cocoa bean, which contains several active compounds responsible for its unique properties.
- The main psychoactive ingredient in chocolate is theobromine, a mild stimulant that can enhance mood and provide a gentle energy boost.
- Dark chocolate also contains small amounts of caffeine, which can contribute to increased alertness and a sense of well-being.

MOOD-ENHANCING COMPOUNDS:

Serotonin: Dark chocolate stimulates the release of serotonin, a neurotransmitter associated with feelings of happiness and well-being. Increased serotonin levels in the brain can help improve mood and reduce symptoms of depression.

Endorphins: Consuming dark chocolate triggers the release of endorphins, the body's natural painkillers, and mood elevators. These endorphins create a sense of pleasure and enhance feelings of contentment and relaxation.

ANTIOXIDANT POWERHOUSE:

- Dark chocolate is packed with antioxidants, particularly flavonoids. These antioxidants help combat oxidative stress, reduce inflammation, and protect brain health.
- The flavonoids in dark chocolate have been linked to improved blood flow and enhanced cognitive function, which can positively impact mood and cognitive performance.

STRESS REDUCTION:

- Dark chocolate has been found to have stress-reducing properties. Consuming a small amount of dark chocolate during stressful situations can help lower stress hormone levels and promote a sense of calmness.
- The combination of its pleasant taste and the release of endorphins and serotonin can provide a soothing effect, aiding in stress management.

HEART-HEALTHY BENEFITS:

- Consuming moderate amounts of dark chocolate, preferably with a high cocoa content (70% or higher), has been associated with several cardiovascular benefits.
- The flavonoids in dark chocolate can improve blood circulation, reduce blood pressure, and decrease the risk of heart disease. A healthy heart is closely linked to improved mood and overall well-being.

MINDFUL INDULGENCE:

- Enjoying dark chocolate mindfully can enhance mood-boosting effects. Take the time to savor the rich flavors, textures, and aromas of dark chocolate.
- Practicing mindful eating allows you to fully appreciate the experience, fostering a sense of relaxation and pleasure.

MODERATION AND QUALITY:

- While dark chocolate offers potential mood-boosting benefits, it is important to consume it in moderation as part of a balanced diet.
- Choose dark chocolate with a high cocoa content and minimal added sugars or unhealthy fats. Opting for organic and fair-trade varieties ensures the highest quality and supports ethical sourcing.

NUTRITIONAL PROFILE

In addition to being a tasty treat, dark chocolate has several nutrients and health advantages. The nutritional profile of dark chocolate is summarized as follows:

MACRONUTRIENTS AND CALORIES:

- An ounce (28 grams) of dark chocolate contains roughly 160–170 calories, making it a caloric-dense food.
- To give it flavor and texture, it contains carbohydrates, including sugars and dietary fiber.
- A moderate amount of fat is also present in dark chocolate, primarily in the form of saturated and monounsaturated fatty acids.

FIBER:

- With 3 grams per ounce, dark chocolate is a good source of dietary fiber.
- Digestive aid, blood sugar regulation, and support for a healthy gut microbiome are all benefits of fiber.

MINERALS:

- Minerals found in dark chocolate include iron, magnesium, copper, and manganese.
- Magnesium supports healthy bones and muscles, while iron is necessary for the body to transport oxygen.
- For several enzymatic reactions in the body, copper and manganese function as cofactors.

ANTIOXIDANTS:

- Flavonoids and polyphenols in particular are abundant in dark chocolate's antioxidant content.
- These substances have strong antioxidant qualities that aid in scavenging free radicals and lowering oxidative stress.
- Due to its higher cocoa content, dark chocolate has higher levels of antioxidants than milk chocolate.

FLAVANOLS:

- Dark chocolate is a good source of flavanols, a type of flavonoid that can be found in cocoa beans.

- Flavanols have been linked to several positive health effects, such as better cardiovascular health, improved cognitive function, and decreased inflammation.

CAFFEINE AND THEOBROMINE:

- Theobromine and caffeine are present in small amounts in dark chocolate.
- Theobromine is a natural stimulant that can give you a little extra energy and possibly improve your mood.
- In moderation, caffeine, another stimulant, can heighten alertness and enhance cognitive function.

GLUCOSE INDEX

- Dark chocolate has a low glycaemic index (GI), making it less likely to raise blood sugar levels than foods high in sugar.
- Dark chocolate contains fiber, good fats, and antioxidants that help slow down the absorption of carbohydrates and lower the glycaemic response.

QUALITY AND COCOA CONTENT:

- Depending on the quality and content of cocoa solids, dark chocolate can have a different nutritional profile.
- Higher cocoa content (70%) and higher quality dark chocolate typically have more antioxidants and fewer added sugar and other additives.
- Due to its high calorie and fat content, dark chocolate should be consumed in moderation. The most nutritional advantages are found in dark chocolate with a higher cocoa content and few added sugars. When incorporating dark chocolate into your diet, keep in mind to take your daily caloric intake and nutritional objectives into account.

LEAFY GREENS

Leafy greens, such as spinach, kale, Swiss chard, and collard greens, are not only rich in essential vitamins and minerals but can also contribute to serotonin production in the body. Exploration of how leafy greens can act as serotonin-boosting foods:

TRYPTOPHAN CONTENT:

- Leafy greens are a source of tryptophan, an essential amino acid that serves as a precursor for serotonin synthesis.
- Tryptophan is converted into 5-hydroxytryptophan (5-HTP), which is further converted into serotonin in the brain.
- While leafy greens may not have as high a tryptophan content as some other protein sources, they still contribute to the overall availability of tryptophan in the body for serotonin production.

FOLATE (VITAMIN B9) CONTENT:

- Leafy greens are excellent sources of folate, also known as vitamin B9.
- Folate plays a crucial role in neurotransmitter synthesis, including serotonin production.
- Serotonin synthesis relies on the enzyme methylenetetrahydrofolate reductase (MTHFR), which requires folate as a cofactor.
- Consuming folate-rich leafy greens supports optimal serotonin production by providing the necessary cofactor for MTHFR.

ANTIOXIDANT CAPACITY:

- Leafy greens are packed with antioxidants, including vitamins C and E, beta-carotene, and various phytochemicals.
- Antioxidants help protect the brain cells and neurotransmitters, including serotonin, from oxidative damage caused by free radicals.

- By reducing oxidative stress, leafy greens support the overall health and function of serotonin-producing neurons.

Magnesium Content:

- Leafy greens are a good source of magnesium, an essential mineral involved in serotonin regulation.
- Magnesium acts as a cofactor for the enzyme tryptophan hydroxylase, which converts tryptophan to 5-HTP, an intermediate in serotonin synthesis.
- Adequate magnesium levels are crucial for optimal serotonin production and function.

FIBER AND BLOOD SUGAR REGULATION:

- Leafy greens are high in dietary fiber, including both soluble and insoluble fiber.
- The fiber content helps regulate blood sugar levels by slowing down the absorption of carbohydrates from the diet.

- Stable blood sugar levels are essential for maintaining steady serotonin production and preventing mood swings associated with blood sugar fluctuations.

NUTRIENT DENSITY:

- Leafy greens are incredibly nutrient-dense, providing a wide array of vitamins and minerals that support overall brain health and mood regulation.
- They contain vitamins such as vitamin C, vitamin K, and several B vitamins (including folate and vitamin B6), which are important for serotonin synthesis and neurotransmitter function.
- Leafy greens also provide minerals like iron, calcium, and potassium, which contribute to optimal brain and nerve function.

ANTI-INFLAMMATORY PROPERTIES:

- Chronic inflammation in the body can negatively impact serotonin levels and overall brain health.

- Leafy greens are known for their anti-inflammatory properties, attributed to the presence of various antioxidants and phytochemicals.
- By reducing inflammation, leafy greens support serotonin production and protect against mood disorders associated with chronic inflammation.

To incorporate leafy greens into your diet as serotonin-boosting foods, consider adding them to salads, soups, smoothies, stir-fries, or as a side dish. Remember to choose fresh, organic options whenever possible to maximize their nutritional benefits. Pairing leafy greens with other serotonin-boosting foods, such as tryptophan-rich proteins or healthy fats, can further enhance serotonin synthesis and support mental well-being.

HEALTH BENEFITS

They provide a wide range of health advantages because they are nutrient-rich. The following are a few of the major health advantages of including leafy greens in your diet:

Leafy greens have a high nutrient density despite having few calories. They are a great source of folate, vitamins A, C, and K. Additionally, they include minerals like calcium, magnesium, and potassium. These nutrients are necessary for many bodily processes, such as blood clotting, bone health, and immune function.

Leafy greens are a rich source of antioxidants, including vitamins C and E, beta-carotene, and several phytonutrients. By defending the body against the oxidative stress brought on by free radicals, antioxidants lower the risk of developing chronic illnesses like heart disease, some cancers, and age-related macular degeneration.

Heart Health: Leafy greens are good for your heart because they contain a variety of nutrients. They contain high levels of dietary nitrates, which have been found to improve blood vessel health and lower blood pressure. Leafy greens' high potassium content helps to maintain normal blood pressure levels.

Leafy greens are a fantastic source of dietary fiber, which is essential for preserving a healthy digestive system. Constipation is avoided, regular bowel movements are encouraged, and the growth of healthy gut bacteria is supported. Additionally, it lowers the risk of digestive diseases like diverticulitis and haemorrhoids and aids in maintaining a healthy weight.

Bone Health: Kale and collard greens, in particular, are abundant in calcium and vitamin K, both of which are crucial for bone health. Calcium is necessary to maintain healthy bones, and vitamin K promotes bone mineralization and controls calcium absorption.

Leafy greens, which contain carotenoids like lutein and zeaxanthin, are good for your eyes. These substances build up in the retina and aid in preventing cataracts and age-related macular degeneration. Another nutrient present in leafy greens, vitamin A, is necessary for healthy vision.

Weight Management: Leafy greens are a great option for weight management because they are high in fiber and low in calories. They give satiety and aid in appetite control, making it simpler to keep a healthy weight. Their high-water content also gives meals more volume without adding too many calories.

Blood Sugar Control: Because leafy greens have a low glycaemic index, their effect on blood sugar levels is negligible. In addition to promoting stable blood sugar levels and lowering the risk of type 2 diabetes, the fiber and other nutrients in leafy greens slow down the digestion and absorption of carbohydrates.

Anti-Inflammatory Properties: Because leafy greens have a high antioxidant content, many of them have anti-inflammatory properties. Numerous illnesses, such as heart disease, diabetes, and some cancers, are linked to chronic inflammation. Consuming leafy greens can support overall health by reducing inflammation.

Culinary Options and Versatility: Leafy greens have a wide range of culinary applications and are incredibly adaptable. They can be used as a nutrient-rich base for wraps and sandwiches, eaten raw in salads, added to smoothies, sautéed, or steamed. You can more successfully add leafy greens to your diet by experimenting with various varieties and recipes.

Leafy greens are a healthy and versatile food that can be enjoyed in many different ways. They can be eaten raw, cooked, or juiced. How to include leafy greens in your diet:

- Add leafy greens to salads.
- Stir-fry leafy greens with vegetables and tofu.
- Make a smoothie with leafy greens, fruit, and yogurt.
- Add leafy greens to soups and stews.
- Make a wrap with leafy greens, hummus, and vegetables.

SALMON

Few foods that are both healthy and delicious can compare to salmon's versatility and health advantages. Salmon is renowned for its many health benefits in addition to being a delectable culinary treat. Its capacity to elevate mood and support mental well-being stands out among its many remarkable qualities. Let's delve into the world of salmon and discover why it is one of the best foods for elevating mood.

Salmon is incredibly high in omega-3 fatty acids, especially eicosapentaenoic acid (EPA) and docosahexaenoic acid (DHA). These essential fatty acids are known to promote mental health and play a significant role in brain function. A diet rich in omega-3 fatty acids has been linked to a decrease in the signs and symptoms of depression, anxiety, and stress, according to numerous studies. The neurotransmitters serotonin and dopamine, which control mood and emotions, are transported by these beneficial fats.

Serotonin, also known as the "feel-good" hormone, is in charge of regulating mood, encouraging happiness, and lowering anxiety. Serotonin production is increased. Tryptophan, an amino acid that is abundant in salmon, is necessary for the brain's production of serotonin. Salmon consumption can naturally increase serotonin levels, enhancing mood and thwarting depressive symptoms.

Vitamin D Boost: Vitamin D, also known as the "sunshine vitamin," is essential for maintaining mood and preventing depression. Salmon is one of the few foods that naturally contain significant amounts of vitamin D, though sunlight is still the main source of this vital vitamin. Salmon is a great option for preserving optimal mental health because one serving can supply a significant amount of the daily recommended intake of this essential nutrient.

B vitamins for Stress Reduction: Salmon is a great source of folate, vitamin B12, vitamin B6, and other B vitamins. These vitamins are necessary for the synthesis of neurotransmitters that regulate mood and reduce stress, such as serotonin and dopamine. Particularly vitamin B12 is well known for promoting brain health and easing depressive symptoms. You can make sure you are getting enough of these stress-relieving B vitamins by including salmon in your diet.

Reducing Inflammation: Several mental health conditions, including depression, have been linked to chronic inflammation in the body. Salmon has strong anti-inflammatory properties because it contains omega-3 fatty acids. These beneficial fats contribute to the reduction of inflammation throughout the body, including the brain, which fosters the best possible mental health.

Salmon is a nutritional powerhouse that not only improves mood but is also a rich source of important nutrients that promote overall health. It is a first-rate source of top-notch protein, which is necessary for the synthesis of neurotransmitters and the synthesis of energy. Salmon also contains plenty of potassium and selenium, two minerals that support blood pressure control and brain health.

Including Salmon in Your Diet: To take advantage of salmon's mood-enhancing properties, think about including it in your weekly menu plan. Salmon can be prepared in a variety of delectable ways, including grilling, baking, and pan-searing. For a balanced, healthy meal, serve it with a side of leafy greens or steamed vegetables. Salmon from a can make a practical addition to salads and sandwiches.

When at all possible, choose wild-caught salmon because it tends to be cleaner and higher in omega-3 fatty acids than farmed salmon. To maximize the mood-enhancing effects of salmon, aim for at least two servings per week.

Because it contains a significant amount of omega-3 fatty acids, which promote brain health and the synthesis of neurotransmitters, salmon stands out as a standout food for elevating mood. It is a nutritional powerhouse due to its natural abundance in the serotonin-boosting amino acid tryptophan, stress-relieving B vitamins, and anti-inflammatory properties.

NUTRITIONAL PROFILE/VALUE OF SALMON

Salmon is a popular fish known for its delicious flavor and numerous health benefits. The nutritional profile of raw, wild-caught Atlantic salmon per 100 grams:

- ❖ Calories: 206 kcal
- ❖ Protein: 22.0 grams
- ❖ Total Fat: 13.4 grams

  - ➢ Saturated Fat: 2.4 grams
  - ➢ Monounsaturated Fat: 4.9 grams
  - ➢ Polyunsaturated Fat: 4.6 grams
- ❖ Cholesterol: 55 milligrams
- ❖ Omega-3 Fatty Acids: 2.3 grams
- ❖ Omega-6 Fatty Acids: 0.8 grams

❖ Vitamin D: 12.5 micrograms (625 IU)
❖ Vitamin B12: 4.9 micrograms
❖ Vitamin B6: 0.6 milligrams
❖ Vitamin A: 162 IU
❖ Niacin: 8.8 milligrams
❖ Thiamine: 0.2 milligrams
❖ Riboflavin: 0.2 milligrams
❖ Pantothenic Acid: 1.2 milligrams
❖ Folate: 13 micrograms
❖ Calcium: 12 milligrams
❖ Iron: 0.9 milligrams
❖ Magnesium: 29 milligrams
❖ Phosphorus: 220 milligrams
❖ Potassium: 410 milligrams
❖ Selenium: 39.8 micrograms
❖ Sodium: 59 milligrams
❖ Zinc: 0.7 milligrams

Please note that the nutritional composition may vary slightly depending on the specific type of salmon and its preparation method. Additionally, farmed salmon may have different nutrient profiles due to differences in diet and living conditions. It's always a good idea to consult specific packaging or reliable sources for accurate and up-to-date information.

HEATH BENEFITS

Rich in Omega-3 Fatty Acids: Salmon is one of the best sources of omega-3 fatty acids, particularly eicosapentaenoic acid (EPA) and docosahexaenoic acid (DHA). These fatty acids have been shown to reduce inflammation, support brain health, and promote heart health. They are also beneficial for reducing the risk of chronic diseases such as heart disease, stroke, and certain types of cancer.

Heart Health: The omega-3 fatty acids found in salmon help to reduce triglyceride levels, lower blood pressure, and decrease the risk of blood clot formation. Regular consumption of salmon has been associated with a reduced risk of heart disease, heart attacks, and strokes.

Brain Function: The omega-3 fatty acids in salmon are essential for brain health and development. They are crucial for maintaining the structure and function of brain cells and can help improve cognitive function, memory, and mood. Some studies have also suggested that omega-3 fatty acids may help reduce the risk of age-related cognitive decline and neurodegenerative diseases such as Alzheimer's disease.

Eye Health: Salmon is a good source of several nutrients that are beneficial for eye health, including omega-3 fatty acids, vitamin D, vitamin A, and the antioxidant astaxanthin. These nutrients help protect the eyes against age-related macular degeneration (AMD) and dry eye syndrome, and they promote overall eye health.

Nutrient-Rich: Salmon is packed with essential nutrients such as high-quality protein, vitamin D, vitamin B12, selenium, and potassium. These nutrients are important for maintaining overall health, supporting the immune system, promoting cell growth and repair, and improving energy levels.

Weight Management: Salmon is a lean source of protein, which can help increase satiety and reduce appetite. Including salmon in your diet can aid in weight management and help you maintain healthy body weight.

Anti-Inflammatory Properties: The omega-3 fatty acids and other bioactive compounds in salmon have anti-inflammatory effects. Regular consumption of salmon may help reduce inflammation in the body, which is associated with various chronic diseases, including heart disease, diabetes, and arthritis.

PINEAPPLE

The tropical fruit pineapple is well-known for its distinctively sweet flavor and bright yellow flesh. In addition to adding flavor to a variety of dishes, pineapple has several healthy ingredients like vitamins, minerals, and enzymes. Tryptophan, an amino acid that is essential for the body's production of serotonin, is one such substance.

A neurotransmitter called serotonin is involved in controlling mood, appetite, sleep, and other vital processes. The "feel-good" neurotransmitter gets its name from the fact that it promotes feelings of joy, relaxation, and general well-being. For maintaining emotional and mental balance, serotonin levels must be adequate.

Tryptophan, a protein-rich food found in pineapple and other foods, is a precursor to the synthesis of serotonin. Our bodies use a variety of enzymes to transform foods containing tryptophan into serotonin after consumption. When compared to other sources like turkey or dairy products, pineapple is not regarded as a high-tryptophan food, but it does contain a moderate amount of the amino acid.

While tryptophan is present in pineapple, compared to other factors affecting serotonin synthesis, it may have a negligible effect on serotonin levels. Other dietary elements, such as the availability of other amino acids and the presence of specific vitamins and minerals, can affect the body's capacity to convert tryptophan into serotonin. In addition, factors like stress, exercise, and sun exposure also affect how serotonin is regulated.

Nevertheless, including pineapple in a healthy diet can boost the production of serotonin in general. Pineapple is a well-liked fruit because of its inherent sweetness and adaptability; it can be consumed in a variety of ways, including as fresh slices, juices, and smoothies, and as an ingredient in dishes like fruit salads and desserts.

It's important to understand that, even though pineapple may help to some extent with serotonin production, it is not a cure or treatment for serotonin-related illnesses like depression or anxiety. Due to the complexity of these conditions, appropriate treatment methods and professional assistance are frequently needed.

To ensure a proper balance of nutrients, it's crucial to maintain a well-rounded diet that includes a variety of foods, just like with any other dietary consideration.

When it comes to mood-boosting foods, pineapples are often overlooked. However, this tropical fruit is not only a delectable and refreshing treat, but it also contains nutrients that contribute to increased serotonin levels in the brain. Serotonin, known as the "feel-good" hormone, plays a vital role in regulating mood, happiness, and overall mental well-being. Reasons why pineapple deserves recognition as one of the serotonin-boosting foods.

RICH IN TRYPTOPHAN:

One of the key components of serotonin production is an amino acid called tryptophan. Tryptophan serves as a precursor to serotonin, meaning the body must produce this important neurotransmitter. Pineapple contains a moderate amount of tryptophan, making it a valuable addition to a serotonin-boosting diet. While pineapple may not have the highest tryptophan, content compared to other foods, it contributes to the overall intake of this essential amino acid.

VITAMIN C CONTENT:

Pineapple is renowned for its high vitamin C content, which provides numerous health benefits. In terms of serotonin production, vitamin C plays a crucial role as it helps convert tryptophan into serotonin in the brain. By consuming pineapple, you are providing your body with an ample supply of vitamin C, which aids in optimizing serotonin synthesis.

BROMELAIN AND MOOD REGULATION:

Another remarkable compound found in pineapples is bromelain, an enzyme with anti-inflammatory properties. While bromelain itself does not directly influence serotonin levels, it contributes to overall well-being by reducing inflammation in the body. Chronic inflammation has been linked to mood disorders such as depression and anxiety, so incorporating pineapple and its bromelain content into your diet may indirectly support a more positive mood and mental health.

HYDRATION AND ENERGY:

Staying hydrated is crucial for maintaining optimal brain function and overall well-being. Pineapple, with its high-water content, can help keep you hydrated throughout the day. Dehydration can lead to fatigue, poor cognitive function, and even mood swings. By including pineapple in your diet, you can help maintain proper hydration levels, which in turn supports serotonin production and a balanced mood.

NATURAL ANTIOXIDANTS:

Pineapple is rich in antioxidants such as vitamin C and beta-carotene, which protect cells from damage caused by harmful free radicals. By reducing oxidative stress, these antioxidants contribute to overall brain health and may indirectly support serotonin production. A healthy brain environment allows for optimal neurotransmitter function and can help maintain stable moods.

TOFU

Popular plant-based protein tofu, which is made from soybeans, is well known for its dietary advantages and a plethora of culinary applications even though tofu does not naturally contain serotonin, the essential amino acids it contains, such as tryptophan, may help the body produce serotonin.

An essential amino acid known as tryptophan functions as a starting point for the production of serotonin. Tryptophan is an amino acid that our bodies use in conjunction with several enzymes to create serotonin when we eat foods containing this amino acid. Along with other high-quality foods rich in protein, including tofu, tryptophan is thought to be present in these foods.

A variety of essential amino acids are provided by including tofu in your diet, which is important for overall health and wellbeing. Tofu typically contains a respectable amount of tryptophan, though the exact amount can vary depending on the brand and preparation. It's important to keep in mind that other dietary components and individual metabolic differences can affect the actual effect of tryptophan on serotonin levels.

Tofu should be eaten with other foods that promote serotonin synthesis in order to maximize any potential serotonin-boosting effects. Included in this are foods high in vitamins and minerals, which help turn tryptophan into serotonin. For instance, magnesium, vitamin C, and vitamin B6 are crucial co-factors in this process.

Tofu can be accompanied by a balanced diet that includes a variety of fruits, vegetables, whole grains, and other protein sources to help support serotonin synthesis. It's important to remember that diet alone cannot treat serotonin-related conditions like depression or anxiety or replace qualified medical care. You must get the right support from a healthcare provider if you are having any mental health issues.

Tofu can be a healthy addition to most diets, but it may not be suitable for people with soy allergies or certain medical conditions, it's also important to note. Before making significant dietary changes or including particular foods for their potential serotonin-boosting effects, it is always advisable to speak with a healthcare provider or registered dietitian.

While tofu does not naturally contain serotonin, the tryptophan it contains can help the body produce serotonin. A well-balanced diet that includes tofu and additional foods that encourage serotonin synthesis can help raise overall serotonin levels.

NUTRITIONAL BENEFITS OF TOFU

High-quality protein: Tofu is an excellent source of protein, making it a valuable option for individuals following vegetarian or vegan diets. It contains all the essential amino acids necessary for the body's protein synthesis.

Low in saturated fat: Tofu is relatively low in saturated fat compared to animal-based protein sources, making it a heart-healthy alternative. Consuming less saturated fat can help lower the risk of heart disease and maintain healthy cholesterol levels.

Low in calories: Tofu is relatively low in calories, making it a suitable food for those looking to manage their weight. It provides a good amount of nutrition without adding excessive calories, especially if prepared using healthy cooking methods.

Source of essential minerals: Tofu contains essential minerals such as calcium, iron, magnesium, phosphorus, and zinc. Calcium is particularly important for maintaining bone health, while iron is necessary for oxygen transport and energy production in the body.

Rich in vitamins: Tofu is a good source of several vitamins, including vitamin E, B vitamins (such as folate, thiamine, and niacin), and vitamin K. Vitamin E is an antioxidant that helps protect cells from damage, while B vitamins are essential for energy metabolism and brain function. Vitamin K plays a vital role in blood clotting and bone health.

Soy isoflavones: Tofu is derived from soybeans, which naturally contain compounds called isoflavones. Isoflavones have been associated with potential health benefits, including reduced risk of heart disease, improved bone health, and relief from menopausal symptoms in some women.

Fiber content: Tofu contains dietary fiber, which aids in digestion and helps maintain healthy blood sugar levels. Fiber also promotes a feeling of fullness, which can be beneficial for weight management.

It's worth noting that the nutritional profile of tofu can vary depending on its preparation method and the type of coagulant used. Additionally, individuals with soy allergies or specific health conditions should consult with their healthcare provider before incorporating tofu into their diet.

EGGS

The humble egg stands out as a serotonin-boosting superstar when it comes to foods that can improve your mood and foster a sense of well-being. The neurotransmitter serotonin, also known as the "feel-good" neurotransmitter, is essential for controlling mood, sleep, and general mental health. Eggs are a delicious and healthy way to support the body's production of serotonin. They are also a rich source of vital nutrients and bioactive compounds. We will examine the exceptional qualities of eggs and how they help to raise serotonin levels.

TRYPTOPHAN: THE SEROTONIN PRECURSOR

Tryptophan, an essential amino acid that is used as a building block for the production of serotonin, is abundant in eggs. The body needs tryptophan to make serotonin because it functions as a precursor to this neurotransmitter. Tryptophan-rich foods, such as eggs, give your brain the raw materials it needs to make this essential neurotransmitter.

B VITAMINS FOR THE SYNTHESIS OF SEROTONIN

In addition to tryptophan, eggs are a good source of B vitamins, especially B6 and B12, which are essential for the synthesis of serotonin. While vitamin B12 aids in maintaining the overall health of the nervous system, vitamin B6 is involved in the conversion of tryptophan into serotonin. By including eggs in your diet, you can make sure that you get enough of these vital B vitamins, which will support the optimal production of serotonin.

CHOLINE: INCREASING SEROTONIN SIGNALLING

Choline, a nutrient recognized for its function in neurotransmitter function, can be found naturally in eggs. Acetylcholine, a neurotransmitter that controls serotonin signalling in the brain, is formed from choline, which functions as its precursor. Choline supports effective neurotransmission, which helps keep serotonin levels balanced and improves mood and emotional wellbeing.

OMEGA-3 FATTY ACIDS: SUPPORT FOR THE BRAIN

The brain's health and serotonin regulation are greatly aided by omega-3 fatty acids, which are primarily found in the yolks of eggs from pasture-raised or omega-3 enriched chickens. Through increased serotonin receptor activity and the promotion of ideal neurotransmitter balance, these healthy fats support the structure and function of brain cells. Omega-3-rich eggs can give you the nutrients you need to support serotonin-related brain functions.

SUNSHINE FOR SEROTONIN: VITAMIN D

Eggs are a great natural source of vitamin D, especially those from chickens that were raised outside. For serotonin synthesis and function, adequate vitamin D levels are essential. Include eggs in your diet to ensure a dietary source of vitamin D, especially during seasons or in areas with limited sunlight. Sunlight exposure aids in the body's production of this essential nutrient.

NUTRITIONAL PROFILE/VALUE

Eggs are highly nutritious and provide a range of essential nutrients. Overview of the nutritional value of eggs:

Protein: Eggs are considered a complete protein source, as they contain all nine essential amino acids needed for protein synthesis in the body. A large egg typically provides around 6 grams of protein, making it an excellent protein-rich food.

Healthy Fats: Eggs contain a good balance of healthy fats, including monounsaturated and polyunsaturated fats. The majority of the fat in eggs is found in the yolk, which also contains essential fat-soluble vitamins.

Vitamins: Eggs are rich in various vitamins, including:

- Vitamin B12: Essential for nerve function, DNA synthesis, and the formation of red blood cells.
- Vitamin B2 (Riboflavin): Important for energy production and the metabolism of fats, carbohydrates, and proteins.

- Vitamin A: Necessary for vision, immune function, and maintaining healthy skin.
- Vitamin D: Promotes calcium absorption, bone health, and immune system function.
- Vitamin E: Acts as an antioxidant and contributes to healthy skin and eyes.
- Vitamin K: Vital for blood clotting and bone health.

Minerals: Eggs are a good source of several essential minerals, including:

- Iron: Important for oxygen transport and preventing iron-deficiency anaemia.
- Phosphorus: Required for bone health, energy production, and various cellular processes.
- Selenium: Acts as an antioxidant and supports thyroid function and immune health.
- Zinc: Necessary for immune function, wound healing, and DNA synthesis.
- Choline: Eggs are an excellent source of choline, an essential nutrient important for brain health, nervous system function, and cell membrane structure.

- Lutein and Zeaxanthin: Eggs contain these antioxidants, which are beneficial for eye health and may help reduce the risk of age-related macular degeneration.

Low in Carbohydrates: Eggs have a minimal carbohydrate content, which makes them suitable for low-carb or ketogenic diets.

It's important to note that the nutritional content of an egg can vary slightly depending on factors such as the chicken's diet and living conditions. Additionally, egg yolks contain cholesterol, so individuals with specific dietary restrictions or conditions should consult with their healthcare provider to determine the appropriate intake.

HEALTH BENEFITS OF EGGS

key health benefits associated with consuming eggs:

Excellent source of high-quality protein: Eggs are considered a complete protein source, meaning they provide all the essential amino acids that the body needs for various functions, including muscle repair, growth, and maintenance.

Rich in essential nutrients: Eggs are packed with essential vitamins and minerals. They are particularly high in vitamin B12, which is crucial for brain function and the production of red blood cells. Eggs also contain vitamins A, D, E, and K, as well as minerals like iron, zinc, selenium, and choline.

Eye health: Eggs contain antioxidants such as lutein and zeaxanthin, which are beneficial for eye health. These compounds may help reduce the risk of age-related macular degeneration and cataracts, two common eye conditions.

Brain function and development: Choline, an essential nutrient found in eggs, plays a vital role in brain function, memory, and development. It is particularly important during pregnancy and early childhood for proper brain development.

Heart health: Contrary to previous beliefs, moderate egg consumption is generally not associated with an increased risk of heart disease for most individuals. Eggs contain healthy unsaturated fats and are a good source of omega-3 fatty acids, which can help reduce inflammation and promote heart health.

Weight management: Eggs are a satisfying and filling food due to their high protein content. Including eggs in your meals can help reduce hunger pangs, control appetite, and aid in weight management.

Nutrient absorption: The fat in eggs helps with the absorption of fat-soluble vitamins such as vitamin A, D, E, and K. Including eggs in your meals can enhance the body's ability to absorb these important nutrients.

TURKEY

We frequently concentrate on the health advantages of the foods we eat. But it's vital to keep in mind that certain foods can also have a significant impact on our mental health. Turkey is one of these foods; it's a delicious, lean protein source that has gained popularity for its capability to raise serotonin levels in the brain. A neurotransmitter called serotonin is well known for its ability to control mood, encourage relaxation, and improve overall mental health. In this article, we'll look at how turkey can help you feel happier and more in control of your emotions.

HOW SEROTONIN CONNECTS:

The neurotransmitter serotonin is frequently referred to as the "feel-good" neurotransmitter due to its link to emotions like happiness, contentment, and wellbeing. The way that it affects mood, sleep, appetite, and even cognitive function is crucial. Serotonin imbalances have been connected to illnesses like depression, anxiety, and insomnia. Turkey enters the picture here.

SEROTONIN AND TRYPTOPHAN:

Tryptophan, an amino acid that serves as a precursor to serotonin, is abundant in turkey. Since tryptophan is an essential amino acid, which means that our bodies cannot naturally produce it, we must get it from food. Once consumed, tryptophan is transformed into serotonin with the aid of particular co-factors and enzymes. We may be able to improve serotonin synthesis by increasing tryptophan availability, which would result in a more steady and upbeat mood.

THE BENEFITS OF TURKEY FOR SEROTONIN BOOST

One of the best dietary sources of tryptophan is turkey, which has a high tryptophan content. The synthesis of serotonin in the brain is based on this amino acid. You can consume more tryptophan by including turkey in your meals, which may cause serotonin levels to rise.

Turkey is a lean protein source that is high in protein and low in fat, making it a wise choice for people trying to eat a diet that is balanced. The synthesis of neurotransmitters, such as serotonin, depends on high-quality protein. Turkey supports serotonin synthesis by supplying the necessary amino acids, enhancing mental performance.

Tryptophan is just one of the important nutrients found in turkey, which also contains a number of other vital nutrients that support overall health. These include vitamins B3 and B6, which help to maintain a healthy nervous system by contributing to the production of serotonin. Turkey also contains minerals like selenium and zinc, which promote cognitive function and aid in oxidative stress protection.

BLOOD SUGAR CONTROL: Turkey helps control blood sugar levels and regulate satiety, in addition to being good for serotonin production. Tryptophan and protein in turkey work together to increase satiety, which lowers the risk of overeating or snacking on unhealthy foods. It's essential to keep blood sugar levels stable if you want to feel alert and happy all day.

INCORPORATING TURKEY INTO YOUR DIET

Consider including turkey in your diet in a variety of ways to maximize its ability to increase serotonin:

Skinless turkey breast is the leanest part of the bird, so choose that instead. It can be grilled, roasted, or sautéed to make a main dish that is high in tryptophan and protein.

Ground turkey is a flexible substitute for beef or pork in dishes like chili, burgers, meatballs, and tacos. For a healthier option, look for lean ground turkey.

Turkey Sandwiches: For a quick and filling meal, use thinly sliced turkey breast in sandwiches or wraps. Fresh vegetables, whole-grain bread, and a source of healthy fats like avocado or hummus should all be included.

Roasted turkey leftovers are delicious when added to salads, stir-fries, or homemade soups. It's a wonderful way to make use of the benefits of the bird while enhancing the flavor and protein of your meals.

In addition to being a delicious and adaptable source of protein, turkey may also improve your mood and mental health. It is a great option for people looking to increase serotonin levels naturally because of its high tryptophan content, nutrient density, and low-fat profile. You can actively support a more stable and optimistic mental state by incorporating turkey into your diet. In order to encourage a happier and healthier you, think about including turkey in your meal plans the next time.

RECIPES USING SEROTONIN-BOOSTING FOODS

BANANA

A diet featuring bananas can contribute to serotonin boosting due to their natural content of tryptophan, which is an essential amino acid involved in serotonin production. Additionally, bananas are a rich source of other nutrients, such as vitamins and minerals, that support overall health and well-being. Here's a sample diet plan that incorporates bananas to help promote serotonin production:

Breakfast:

Banana and Almond Butter Smoothie: Blend a ripe banana, a tablespoon of almond butter, a cup of almond milk, and a handful of spinach. This smoothie provides a combination of tryptophan from the banana, healthy fats from almond butter, and vitamins from spinach.

Mid-Morning Snack:

Banana and Greek Yogurt: Enjoy a small container of Greek yogurt topped with sliced bananas. Greek yogurt is high in protein, which supports the synthesis of serotonin, while bananas provide tryptophan and additional vitamins and minerals.

Lunch:

Grilled Chicken and Banana Salad: Prepare a salad with grilled chicken breast, mixed greens, cherry tomatoes, cucumber slices, and sliced bananas. Top it with a light dressing made from olive oil, lemon juice, and a dash of honey.

Afternoon Snack:

Banana and Nut Mix: Combine a small, ripe banana with a handful of mixed nuts, such as almonds, walnuts, and cashews. Nuts provide healthy fats and protein, while the banana adds natural sweetness and tryptophan.

Dinner:

Baked Salmon with Banana Salsa: Season a salmon fillet with herbs and bake it until cooked through. Serve it with a fresh salsa made from diced bananas, tomatoes, red onion, cilantro, lime juice, and a pinch of salt. This dish provides a balance of protein, omega-3 fatty acids, and tryptophan.

Evening Snack:

Banana and Dark Chocolate: Dip slices of banana into melted dark chocolate and let them cool in the refrigerator until the chocolate hardens. Dark chocolate contains antioxidants and can enhance mood, while the banana adds natural sweetness and tryptophan.

It's important to note that while bananas can contribute to serotonin production, they are not the sole factor influencing serotonin levels. A well-rounded diet, regular physical activity, adequate sleep, and managing stress are all crucial for maintaining optimal serotonin levels and overall mental well-being.

Additionally, individual dietary needs and preferences may vary, so feel free to modify the suggested meal plan based on your specific requirements.

Bananas are a delightful fruit known for their natural sweetness and versatility in various dishes. They are not only a tasty snack but can also contribute to serotonin production due to their high levels of tryptophan and other essential nutrients.

RECIPES FEATURING BANANAS

Banana and Almond Butter Smoothie:

Ingredients:

- 2 ripe bananas
- 2 tablespoons almond butter
- 1 cup almond milk (or your preferred plant-based milk)
- 1 tablespoon honey or maple syrup (optional)
- A sprinkle of cinnamon (optional)
- Ice cubes (optional)

Instructions:

1. Peel the bananas and place them in a blender.
2. Add almond butter, almond milk, honey or maple syrup (if desired), and cinnamon (if using).
3. Blend until smooth and creamy.
4. If desired, add a few ice cubes and blend again until well combined.
5. Pour into a glass and enjoy this delicious and serotonin-boosting smoothie.

Banana Oatmeal Pancakes:

Ingredients:

- 1 ripe banana, mashed
- 1 cup rolled oats
- 1/2 cup milk (dairy or plant-based)
- 1 egg (or flaxseed egg for a vegan option)
- 1 tablespoon honey or maple syrup
- 1/2 teaspoon vanilla extract
- 1/2 teaspoon baking powder
- Pinch of salt
- Coconut oil or cooking spray for greasing

Instructions:

1. In a mixing bowl, combine the mashed banana, rolled oats, milk, egg (or flaxseed egg), honey or maple syrup, vanilla extract, baking powder, and salt. Mix well until all the ingredients are thoroughly combined.

2. Heat a non-stick skillet or griddle over medium heat and lightly grease it with coconut oil or cooking spray.

3. Pour approximately 1/4 cup of the pancake batter onto the skillet for each pancake.

4. Cook for 2-3 minutes until bubbles form on the surface, then flip the pancake and cook for an additional 2-3 minutes until golden brown.

5. Repeat the process with the remaining batter.

6. Serve the pancakes with sliced bananas, a drizzle of honey or maple syrup, and a sprinkle of cinnamon, if desired.

Grilled Banana with Dark Chocolate:

Ingredients:

- 2 ripe bananas
- 2 tablespoons dark chocolate chips or chopped dark chocolate
- 1 tablespoon chopped nuts (such as almonds, walnuts, or pecans)
- Honey or maple syrup for drizzling (optional)

Instructions:

1. Preheat the grill to medium heat.
2. Leave the bananas unpeeled and make a lengthwise slit along the inside curve of each banana, being careful not to cut through the skin.
3. Stuff the slit with dark chocolate chips or chopped dark chocolate and sprinkle with chopped nuts.
4. Place the bananas on the grill, slit-side up, and cook for 5-7 minutes until the chocolate is melted and the bananas are softened.
5. Remove the bananas from the grill and let them cool slightly.

6. Peel the bananas and serve them warm, drizzled
    with honey or maple syrup if desired.

These recipes offer delicious and creative ways to
incorporate bananas into your diet while enjoying their
serotonin-boosting benefits. Whether it's a refreshing
smoothie, a comforting pancake breakfast, or a delightful
grilled dessert, bananas can contribute to your overall well-
being and uplift your mood.

NUTS AND SEEDS

A diet featuring nuts and seeds can be beneficial for serotonin boosting due to their high content of tryptophan, which is an essential amino acid involved in serotonin production. Additionally, nuts and seeds are excellent sources of healthy fats, fiber, and other nutrients that support overall health. Here's a sample diet plan that incorporates nuts and seeds to help promote serotonin production:

BREAKFAST:

Overnight Chia Pudding: In a jar, combine 2 tablespoons of chia seeds, 1 cup of almond milk, a teaspoon of honey or maple syrup, and a sprinkle of cinnamon. Mix well and let it sit in the refrigerator overnight. In the morning, top the pudding with a handful of mixed nuts, such as almonds, walnuts, and cashews.

MID-MORNING SNACK:

Trail Mix: Prepare a small bag of trail mix containing a mix of your favorite nuts and seeds, such as almonds, pumpkin seeds, sunflower seeds, and dried cranberries or raisins. This snack provides a combination of healthy fats, fiber, and tryptophan.

LUNCH:

Quinoa and Mixed Nut Salad: Cook quinoa according to package instructions and let it cool. In a bowl, combine cooked quinoa, a handful of mixed greens, cherry tomatoes, cucumber slices, and a variety of nuts, such as pistachios, pecans, and pine nuts. Drizzle with a simple dressing made from olive oil, lemon juice, and a touch of honey.

AFTERNOON SNACK:

Nut Butter and Apple Slices: Spread a tablespoon of your favorite nut butter, such as almond or cashew butter, on apple slices. Apples provide fiber while nut butter adds healthy fats and tryptophan.

DINNER:

Roasted Salmon with Sesame Seeds: Season a salmon fillet with your preferred herbs and spices and roast it in the oven until cooked through. Sprinkle the salmon with toasted sesame seeds before serving. Serve it with a side of steamed vegetables and quinoa or brown rice.

Evening Snack:

Greek Yogurt with Flaxseeds: Enjoy a small cup of Greek yogurt topped with a tablespoon of ground flaxseeds and a drizzle of honey. Flaxseeds are an excellent source of omega-3 fatty acids, fiber, and tryptophan.

RECIPES FEATURING NUTS AND SEEDS

Incorporating nuts and seeds into your diet can provide a variety of nutrients, including tryptophan, which can contribute to serotonin production. Here's a delicious recipe that features nuts and seeds to help boost serotonin levels:

Warm Quinoa Salad with Nuts and Seeds:

Ingredients:

- 1 cup cooked quinoa
- 1 tablespoon olive oil

- 1 small red onion, thinly sliced
- 2 cloves garlic, minced
- 1 red bell pepper, diced
- 1 cup cherry tomatoes, halved
- 1 cup baby spinach
- ¼ cup chopped nuts (such as almonds, walnuts, or cashews)
- 2 tablespoons mixed seeds (such as pumpkin seeds, sunflower seeds, or sesame seeds)
- Juice of 1 lemon
- Salt and pepper to taste

Instructions:

1. Heat olive oil in a large skillet over medium heat. Add the red onion and garlic, and sauté until the onion becomes translucent.
2. Add the red bell pepper to the skillet and cook for a few minutes until slightly softened. Then, add the cherry tomatoes and cook for another 2-3 minutes.
3. Stir in the cooked quinoa and baby spinach, allowing the spinach to wilt. Cook for an additional 2-3 minutes to warm through.

4. In a separate dry pan, toast the chopped nuts and mixed seeds over low heat for a few minutes until lightly golden and fragrant.
5. Remove both pans from heat. Combine the toasted nuts and seeds with the quinoa mixture.
6. Squeeze the lemon juice over the salad and season with salt and pepper to taste. Toss everything together until well combined.
7. Serve the warm quinoa salad in bowls and enjoy as a nutrient-packed serotonin-boosting meal.

Roasted Salmon with Sesame Seeds:

Ingredients:

- 2 fillets of salmon
- Sesame oil, two tablespoons
- 2/fourths cup soy sauce
- 1 tablespoon of maple syrup or honey
- 2 minced garlic cloves
- a serving of sesame seeds
- pepper and salt as desired
- (Optional) Garnish: fresh cilantro or green onions

Instructions:

1. Turn on the oven to 400 °F (200 °C). To keep things from sticking, line a baking sheet with parchment paper or lightly grease it.
2. Mix the sesame oil, soy sauce, honey or maple syrup, minced garlic, salt, and pepper in a small bowl.
3. Place the salmon fillets skin-side down on the prepared baking sheet. With some of the sesame oil mixture set aside for later, generously brush the tops of the fillets.
4. Over the salmon fillets, evenly distribute the sesame seeds and lightly press them into place.
5. Roast the salmon in the preheated oven for about 12-15 minutes, or until it flakes easily with a fork and reaches your desired level of doneness.
6. To add more flavor, take the salmon out of the oven and drizzle it with the remaining sesame oil mixture.
7. If desired, garnish with green onions or fresh cilantro.
8. Serve the sesame-seed roasted salmon hot with steamed vegetables, rice, or a crisp salad.

You can customize this recipe by adding other vegetables, herbs, or spices according to your taste preferences. Feel free to experiment and make it your own!

Remember that while incorporating nuts and seeds into your diet can support serotonin production, it's important to maintain a balanced and varied diet along with other healthy lifestyle practices to promote optimal mental well-being.

DARK CHOCOLATE

Dark chocolate is often associated with a positive impact on mood and serotonin levels due to its content of antioxidants, minerals, and bioactive compounds. Here's a recipe that incorporates dark chocolate to potentially support serotonin production:

RECIPE FEATURING DARK CHOCOLATE

Dark Chocolate and Berry Parfait

Ingredients:

- 1 cup Greek yogurt
- 1 tablespoon honey or maple syrup
- 1 teaspoon vanilla extract
- ½ cup mixed berries (such as strawberries, blueberries, and raspberries)
- 1 ounce (about 30 grams) dark chocolate, chopped
- 2 tablespoons chopped nuts (such as almonds or walnuts)
- Fresh mint leaves (for garnish, optional)

Instructions:

1. In a bowl, combine Greek yogurt, honey or maple syrup, and vanilla extract. Mix well until smooth.
2. In serving glasses or bowls, layer the yogurt mixture, mixed berries, chopped dark chocolate, and nuts. Repeat the layers until all the ingredients are used.
3. Finish with a sprinkle of chopped nuts and a garnish of fresh mint leaves, if desired.
4. Place the parfaits in the refrigerator for at least 30 minutes to allow the flavors to meld together.
5. Serve chilled and enjoy as a serotonin-boosting dessert or snack.

Dark Chocolate Banana Smoothie

Ingredients:

- 1 ripe banana
- 1 cup almond milk (or any other type of milk)
- 2 tablespoons dark chocolate chips or grated dark chocolate
- 1 tablespoon of optionally more honey or maple syrup

- 1/2 teaspoon vanilla extract
- Ice cubes

Instructions:

1. Peel the banana and place it in a blender.
2. Add almond milk, dark chocolate chips or grated dark chocolate, honey or maple syrup (if using), vanilla extract, and a handful of ice cubes.
3. until creamy and smooth, blend at high speed.
4. Pour into a glass and enjoy this delicious and serotonin-boosting dark chocolate banana smoothie!

Dark Chocolate Trail Mix

Ingredients:

- 1 cup raw almonds
- 1 cup pumpkin seeds
- 1 cup dried cranberries
- 1/2 cup dark chocolate chunks or chips
- 1/2 cup unsweetened coconut flakes

Instructions:

1. In a large mixing bowl, combine raw almonds, pumpkin seeds, dried cranberries, dark chocolate chunks or chips, and unsweetened coconut flakes.
2. Toss everything together until well mixed.
3. A snack bag or sealed container should be used to transfer the trail mix.
4. Grab a handful whenever you need a serotonin-boosting and energizing snack!

Dark Chocolate Oatmeal

Ingredients:

- 1 cup rolled oats
- 2 cups water
- Pinch of salt
- 2 tablespoons dark cocoa powder
- 2 tablespoons dark chocolate chips or grated dark chocolate
- 1 tablespoon of optionally more honey or maple syrup

- Sliced bananas or berries for topping (optional)

Instructions:

1. Bring water to a rolling boil in a medium saucepan. Put a dash of salt in.
2. Turn the heat down to medium-low after stirring in the rolled oats. The oats should be cooked for about 5 minutes, stirring occasionally, until thick.
3. Add dark cocoa powder, dark chocolate chips or grated dark chocolate, and honey or maple syrup (if using). Stir until the chocolate is melted and well incorporated.
4. Take it off the fire and give it a minute or two to cool.
5. Serve the dark chocolate oatmeal in bowls and top with sliced bananas or berries, if desired. Enjoy a warm and serotonin-boosting breakfast!

Dark Chocolate Avocado Mousse

Ingredients:

- 2 ripe avocados

- 1/4 cup dark cocoa powder
- 1/4 cup maple syrup or agave nectar
- 1 teaspoon vanilla extract
- Pinch of salt
- Dark chocolate shavings for garnish (optional)

Instructions:

1. Avocados should be cut in half, the pits taken out, and the flesh scooped into a food processor or blender.
2. Add dark cocoa powder, maple syrup or agave nectar, vanilla extract, and a pinch of salt.
3. Blend until emulsified and creamy, stopping to scrape down the sides as necessary.
4. Transfer the mousse to serving bowls or glasses.
5. If desired, garnish with dark chocolate shavings.
6. To help the mousse firm, place it in the refrigerator for at least 30 minutes.
7. Indulge in this rich and serotonin-boosting dark chocolate avocado mousse!

Dark chocolate contains compounds like flavonoids, which have been associated with potential mood-boosting effects.

The combination of dark chocolate, Greek yogurt, berries, and nuts provides a balance of nutrients, including tryptophan, antioxidants, healthy fats, and protein. These ingredients together can contribute to serotonin production and support overall well-being.

Remember to choose dark chocolate with a high cocoa content (70% or more) for the most health benefits. However, moderation is key, as dark chocolate is still calorie-dense. Enjoy this parfait as part of a balanced diet and consult with a healthcare professional or registered dietitian for personalized advice based on your specific dietary needs and health considerations.

LEAFY GREENS

RECIPES FEATURING LEAFY GREENS

Spinach and Feta Stuffed Mushrooms

Ingredients:

- 12 large mushrooms
- 2 cups fresh spinach, chopped
- 1/2 cup feta cheese, crumbled
- 2 cloves garlic, minced
- 1 tablespoon olive oil
- Salt and pepper to taste

Instructions:

1. Bake at 375°F (190°C) for 15 minutes with a baking sheet lined with parchment paper.
2. The mushroom stems should be cut off and stored separately. The prepared baking sheet should now have the mushroom caps on it.
3. Olive oil is heated in a skillet at a medium temperature. Sauté garlic till aromatic after adding.

4. Cook the spinach until it wilts after being added. Take it off the fire and give it a minute to cool.
5. In a bowl, combine the cooked spinach, crumbled feta cheese, salt, and pepper. Mix well.
6. Stuff each mushroom cap with the spinach and feta mixture.
7. Place the stuffed mushrooms on the baking sheet and bake for about 15-20 minutes, or until the mushrooms are tender and the filling is lightly golden.
8. Serve as an appetizer or side dish for a serotonin-boosting meal.

Kale and Quinoa Salad

Ingredients:

- 2 cups kale, chopped
- 1 cup cooked quinoa
- 1/4 cup dried cranberries
- 1/4 cup chopped walnuts
- 1/4 cup crumbled goat cheese
- 2 tablespoons lemon juice
- 2 tablespoons olive oil

- Salt and pepper to taste

Instructions:

1. Combine chopped kale, cooked quinoa, chopped walnuts, crumbled goat cheese, dried cranberries, and them in a big bowl.
2. In a small bowl, combine the lemon juice, olive oil, salt, and pepper.
3. Toss the salad to combine the dressing after adding it.
4. The salad will taste better if the flavors have chance to meld together.
5. Serve as a refreshing and serotonin-boosting salad.

Swiss Chard Stir-Fry

Ingredients:

- 1 bunch of Swiss chard, cut after separating the stems and leaves.
- 1 bell pepper, thinly sliced
- 1 onion, thinly sliced
- 2 cloves garlic, minced

- 1 tablespoon soy sauce
- 1 tablespoon sesame oil
- 1 tablespoon rice vinegar
- 1 teaspoon honey or maple syrup (optional)
- Sesame seeds for garnish (optional)

Instructions:

1. Large skillet or wok over medium heat, add sesame oil.
2. Add minced garlic and sauté until fragrant.
3. Add sliced onion and bell pepper to the skillet and stir-fry for a few minutes until they begin to soften.
4. Add chopped Swiss chard stems and continue to stir-fry for another 2-3 minutes.
5. Swiss chard leaves should be added and cooked until wilted.
6. In a small bowl, whisk together soy sauce, rice vinegar, and honey or maple syrup (if using).
7. Pour the sauce over the stir-fried vegetables and toss to coat evenly.
8. Allow the ingredients to melt together by cooking for one more minute.
9. Garnish with sesame seeds, if desired.

10. Serve as a delicious and serotonin-boosting side dish.

Broccoli and Spinach Soup

Ingredients:

- 2 cups broccoli florets
- 2 cups fresh spinach leaves
- 1 onion, chopped
- 2 cloves garlic, minced
- 4 cups vegetable broth
- 1 tablespoon olive oil
- Salt and pepper to taste

Instructions:

1. In a big pot, heat up the olive oil over medium heat.
2. Add chopped onion and minced garlic. Sauté until translucent.
3. Add broccoli florets and vegetable broth to the pot. Bring to a boil and let it simmer for about 10 minutes or until the broccoli is tender.

4. Add fresh spinach leaves and cook for an additional 2-3 minutes until wilted.
5. To purée the soup until it is smooth and creamy, either use an immersion blender or transfer it to a blender.
6. Season with salt and pepper to taste.
7. Serve the broccoli and spinach soup hot, and enjoy its serotonin-boosting benefits.

Collard Greens and Chickpea Curry

Ingredients:

- 1 bunch sliced collard greens with the stems removed.
- 1 can chickpeas, drained and rinsed
- 1 onion, chopped
- 2 cloves garlic, minced
- 1 can coconut milk
- 2 tablespoons curry powder
- 1 tablespoon olive oil
- Salt and pepper to taste
- Cooked rice for serving

Instructions:

1. Over medium heat, warm the olive oil in a sizable saucepan or skillet.
2. Add minced garlic and onion, chopped. Sauté until the onion is transparent and aromatic.
3. Add curry powder and stir for about a minute until fragrant.
4. Add chopped collard greens and cook for a few minutes until wilted.
5. Stir in the chickpeas and coconut milk. Season with salt and pepper.
6. Simmer for about 15-20 minutes, allowing the flavors to meld together and the collard greens to become tender.
7. Serve the collard greens and chickpea curry over cooked rice for a hearty and serotonin-boosting meal.

SALMON

RECIPES FEATURING SALMON

Lemon Garlic Baked Salmon

Ingredients:

- 4 salmon fillets
- 2 tablespoons olive oil
- 2 cloves garlic, minced
- Zest and juice of 1 lemon
- Salt and pepper to taste
- Fresh parsley, chopped (for garnish)

Instructions:

1. Bake at 375°F (190°C) for 15 minutes with a baking sheet lined with parchment paper.
2. On the baking sheet, arrange the salmon fillets.
3. Olive oil, minced garlic, lemon zest, lemon juice, salt, and pepper should all be combined in a small bowl.

4. The salmon fillets are equally coated after being brushed with the mixture.
5. For about 12 to 15 minutes, or until the salmon is cooked through and flakes readily with a fork, bake in the preheated oven.
6. After taking it out of the oven, top it with fresh parsley.
7. For a supper that will increase serotonin levels, serve the lemon-garlic baked salmon with your favorite side dishes.

Teriyaki Glazed Salmon

Ingredients:

- 4 salmon fillets
- 1/4 cup low-sodium soy sauce
- 2 tablespoons honey or maple syrup
- 1 tablespoon rice vinegar
- 2 cloves garlic, minced
- 1 teaspoon grated fresh ginger
- Sesame seeds for garnish (optional)
- Sliced green onions for garnish (optional)

Instructions:

1. To make the teriyaki glaze, combine soy sauce, honey or maple syrup, rice vinegar, chopped garlic, and grated ginger in a bowl.
2. Put the salmon fillets in a zip-top bag or shallow dish and cover them with the teriyaki glaze. Refrigerate the salmon for at least 30 minutes to let it marinade.
3. Preheating the grill or grill pan to medium-high heat is recommended.
4. Remove the salmon from the marinade and discard the excess.
5. Grill the salmon for about 4-5 minutes per side, or until cooked to your desired level of doneness.
6. If desired, add sesame seeds and thinly sliced green onions as a garnish.
7. Serve the teriyaki glazed salmon with steamed vegetables or rice for a serotonin-boosting and flavorful meal.

Salmon and Quinoa Salad

Ingredients:

- 2 salmon fillets

- 1 cup cooked quinoa
- 2 cups mixed greens
- 1 cucumber, diced
- 1 bell pepper, diced
- 1/4 cup cherry tomatoes, halved
- 1/4 cup sliced red onion
- Lemon vinaigrette dressing:
- 2 tablespoons olive oil
- Juice of 1 lemon
- 1 tablespoon Dijon mustard
- Salt and pepper to taste

Instructions:

1. Bake at 375°F (190°C) for 15 minutes with a baking sheet lined with parchment paper.
2. Add salt and pepper to the salmon fillets before placing them on the baking sheet.
3. For about 12 to 15 minutes, or until the salmon is cooked through and flakes readily with a fork, bake in the preheated oven.
4. Take the salmon out of the oven and allow it to cool slightly.

5. In a large bowl, combine cooked quinoa, mixed greens, diced cucumber, diced bell pepper, halved cherry tomatoes, and sliced red onion.

6. In a small bowl, whisk together olive oil, lemon juice, Dijon mustard, salt, and pepper to make the lemon vinaigrette dressing.

7. Flake the baked salmon into chunks and add it to the salad.

8. Drizzle the lemon vinaigrette dressing over the salad and toss to combine.

9. Serve the salmon and quinoa salad as a serotonin-boosting and nutritious meal.

Herb-Crusted Salmon

Ingredients:

- 4 salmon fillets
- 1/4 cup fresh parsley, chopped
- 2 tablespoons fresh dill, chopped
- 2 tablespoons fresh chives, chopped
- 2 tablespoons grated Parmesan cheese
- 2 tablespoons olive oil
- Salt and pepper to taste

- Lemon wedges for serving

Instructions:

1. A baking sheet should be lined with parchment paper and the oven should be preheated to 425°F (220°C).
2. In a bowl, combine chopped parsley, dill, chives, grated Parmesan cheese, olive oil, salt, and pepper to make the herb crust mixture.
3. The salmon fillets should be placed on the prepared baking sheet.
4. Press the herb crust mixture onto the top of each salmon fillet, coating them evenly.
5. Bake in the preheated oven for about 12-15 minutes, or until the salmon is cooked through and the herb crust is golden brown.
6. Take it out of the oven, then let it to cool.
7. Serve the herb-crusted salmon with lemon wedges for squeezing over the top. Enjoy a flavorful and serotonin-boosting meal.

Salmon Tacos with Avocado Salsa

Ingredients:

- 4 salmon fillets
- 1 teaspoon chili powder
- 1/2 teaspoon ground cumin
- 1/2 teaspoon paprika
- Salt and pepper to taste
- 8 small flour tortillas
- Avocado salsa:
- 1 ripe avocado, diced
- 1/4 cup diced red onion
- 1/4 cup chopped fresh cilantro
- Juice of 1 lime
- Salt and pepper to taste

Instructions:

1. The grill or grill pan should be preheated to medium-high heat.
2. In a small bowl, combine chili powder, cumin, paprika, salt, and pepper to make the spice rub.

3. Season the salmon fillets with the spice rub, coating them evenly.
4. Grill the salmon fillets for about 4-5 minutes per side, or until cooked to your desired level of doneness.
5. Remove from the grill and let the salmon cool slightly. Flake into chunks.
6. In a separate bowl, combine diced avocado, diced red onion, chopped cilantro, lime juice, salt, and pepper to make the avocado salsa.
7. The flour tortillas should be warmed as directed on the packaging.
8. Assemble the tacos by placing a portion of the flaked salmon on each tortilla, and top with avocado salsa.
9. Serve the salmon tacos as a serotonin-boosting and delicious meal.

TURKEY

RECIPE FEATURING TURKEY

Turkey and Vegetable Stir-Fry

Ingredients:

- Sliced into thin strips, 1 pound of turkey breast
- 2 cups of a variety of veggies, such as carrots, broccoli, and bell peppers
- 2 cloves garlic, minced
- 2 tablespoons low-sodium soy sauce
- 1 tablespoon sesame oil
- 1 tablespoon honey or maple syrup
- 1/2 teaspoon grated fresh ginger
- Salt and pepper to taste
- Cooked brown rice or quinoa for serving

Instructions:

1. In a sizable skillet or wok, warm the sesame oil over medium-high heat.
2. Add grated ginger and minced garlic to the skillet. Sauté until aromatic for about a minute.

3. Add the turkey breast strips and heat thoroughly until browned.
4. The mixed vegetables should be crisp-tender after a few minutes of stir-frying in the skillet.
5. In a small bowl, whisk together low-sodium soy sauce, honey or maple syrup, salt, and pepper.
6. Pour the sauce over the turkey and vegetables in the skillet. Stir well to coat everything evenly.
7. Cook for another minute or two until the sauce thickens slightly.
8. Serve the turkey and vegetable stir-fry over cooked brown rice or quinoa for a serotonin-boosting and satisfying meal.

Turkey and Kale Salad

Ingredients:

- 1-pound turkey breast, cooked and shredded
- 4 cups kale, chopped
- 1 cup cherry tomatoes, halved
- 1/2 cup sliced cucumber
- 1/4 cup sliced red onion
- 1/4 cup crumbled feta cheese

- 2 tablespoons lemon juice
- 2 tablespoons olive oil
- Salt and pepper to taste

Instructions:

1. In a large bowl, combine chopped kale, cherry tomatoes, sliced cucumber, sliced red onion, and crumbled feta cheese.
2. To create the dressing, combine the lemon juice, olive oil, salt, and pepper in a small bowl.
3. To the salad, add the chopped turkey breast.
4. Over the salad, drizzle the dressing and toss to blend.
5. Allowing time for the flavors to mingle together will help the salad taste better.
6. Serve the turkey and kale salad as a serotonin-boosting and nutritious meal.

Turkey and Quinoa Stuffed Peppers

Ingredients:

- 4 bell peppers
- 1-pound ground turkey
- 1 cup cooked quinoa
- 1/2 cup diced tomatoes
- 1/2 cup diced zucchini
- 1/4 cup diced onion
- 2 cloves garlic, minced
- 1 teaspoon dried basil
- 1 teaspoon dried oregano
- Salt and pepper to taste
- Shredded mozzarella cheese for topping (optional)

Instructions:

1. Prepare a baking dish with grease and preheat the oven to 375°F (190°C).
2. The bell peppers' tops should be cut off so the seeds and membranes can be removed.
3. In a large skillet, cook the ground turkey over medium heat until browned.

4. Add diced tomatoes, diced zucchini, diced onion, minced garlic, dried basil, dried oregano, salt, and pepper to the skillet. Cook for a few minutes until the vegetables are softened.
5. Add the cooked quinoa and mix thoroughly.
6. Stuff the bell peppers with the turkey and quinoa mixture and place them in the greased baking dish.
7. If preferred, top each stuffed pepper with shredded mozzarella cheese.
8. Bake in the preheated oven for about 25-30 minutes, or until the peppers are tender and the cheese is melted and golden.
9. Remove from the oven and let the stuffed peppers cool slightly before serving.
10. Enjoy the turkey and quinoa stuffed peppers as a serotonin-boosting and flavorful meal.

Turkey and Spinach Wrap

Ingredients:

- 1 pound of cooked and thinly sliced turkey breast
- 4 large whole wheat tortillas
- 1 cup fresh spinach leaves

- 1/2 cup sliced avocado
- 1/4 cup sliced red onion
- 1/4 cup Greek yogurt or hummus
- Salt and pepper to taste

Instructions:

1. Lay out the whole wheat tortillas on a clean surface.
2. Spread Greek yogurt or hummus evenly over each tortilla.
3. Place a layer of fresh spinach leaves on top of the yogurt or hummus.
4. Arrange the sliced turkey breast, sliced avocado, and sliced red onion over the spinach.
5. Sprinkle salt and pepper to taste over the filling.
6. Each tortilla should be securely rolled, with the sides tucked in as you go.
7. Serve the wraps by cutting them in half diagonally.
8. Enjoy the turkey and spinach wraps as a serotonin-boosting and convenient meal.

Turkey and Sweet Potato Chili

Ingredients:

- 1-pound ground turkey
- 1 sweet potato, peeled and diced
- 1 onion, diced
- 2 cloves garlic, minced
- 1 can diced tomatoes
- 1 can kidney beans, drained and rinsed
- 2 tablespoons chili powder
- 1 teaspoon cumin
- 1 teaspoon paprika
- Salt and pepper to taste
- Fresh cilantro, chopped (for garnish)

Instructions:

1. Cook the ground turkey until browned over medium heat in a big saucepan or Dutch oven.
2. Add diced sweet potato, diced onion, and minced garlic to the pot. Cook for a few minutes until the onion is translucent and the sweet potato starts to soften.

3. Stir in the diced tomatoes, kidney beans, chili powder, cumin, paprika, salt, and pepper.
4. When the sweet potato is fork-tender and the flavors are well-balanced, bring the chili to a simmer and let it stew for approximately 20 to 25 minutes.
5. If necessary, adjust the seasoning.
6. Serve the turkey and sweet potato chili hot, garnished with fresh cilantro.
7. Enjoy the chili as a serotonin-boosting and comforting meal.

EGGS

RECIPE FEATURING EGGS

Veggie Omelette

Ingredients:

- 3 eggs
- 1/4 cup chopped bell peppers (any color)
- 1/4 cup chopped onion
- 1/4 cup sliced mushrooms
- 1/4 cup chopped spinach
- Salt and pepper to taste
- 1 tablespoon olive oil
- Grated cheese (optional)

Instructions:

1. Beat the eggs in a bowl and season with salt and pepper.
2. In a non-stick skillet, warm up the olive oil over medium heat.
3. Add bell peppers, onion, mushrooms, and spinach to the skillet. Sauté until the vegetables are softened.

4. Pour the beaten eggs into the skillet, spreading them evenly over the vegetables.
5. Cook for a few minutes until the edges of the omelette start to set.
6. If desired, sprinkle grated cheese over the omelette.
7. Carefully fold the omelette in half and cook for another minute or until the eggs are fully set.
8. Serve the veggie omelette hot, and enjoy its serotonin-boosting benefits.

Avocado and Egg Toast

Ingredients:

- 2 slices whole wheat bread
- 1 ripe avocado
- 2 eggs
- Salt and pepper to taste
- Red pepper flakes (optional)
- Fresh cilantro or parsley (for garnish)

Instructions:

1. The whole wheat bread pieces should be toasted until golden brown.
2. Remove the pit by halves the avocado. Take the flesh out and mash it with a fork until it is smooth.
3. Spread the mashed avocado evenly on the toasted bread slices.
4. Heat a non-stick skillet over medium heat and crack the eggs into the skillet.
5. Cook the eggs to your desired level of doneness (e.g., fried, sunny-side-up, or poached).
6. Season the eggs with salt, pepper, and red pepper flakes, if desired.
7. Carefully place one cooked egg on top of each avocado toast.
8. Garnish with fresh cilantro or parsley.
9. Serve the avocado and egg toast for a serotonin-boosting breakfast or brunch.

Spinach and Feta Scrambled Eggs

Ingredients:

- 4 eggs
- 1 cup fresh spinach leaves

- 1/4 cup crumbled feta cheese
- 2 tablespoons milk
- Salt and pepper to taste
- 1 tablespoon olive oil

Instructions:

1. Whisk the eggs, milk, salt, and pepper in a bowl.
2. The olive oil should be heated in a skillet over medium heat.
3. Add the spinach leaves to the skillet and sauté until wilted.
4. Pour the beaten eggs into the skillet, stirring gently with a spatula.
5. Continue stirring the eggs until they start to set.
6. Sprinkle the crumbled feta cheese over the eggs and continue cooking until the eggs are fully cooked and the cheese is melted.
7. Remove from heat and let the scrambled eggs sit for a minute.
8. Serve the spinach and feta scrambled eggs warm, and enjoy their serotonin-boosting properties.

Egg Salad Lettuce Wraps

Ingredients:

- 4 hard-boiled eggs, chopped
- 1/4 cup mayonnaise
- 1 tablespoon Dijon mustard
- 1 stalk celery, diced
- 2 tablespoons chopped fresh dill
- Salt and pepper to taste
- Large lettuce leaves (such as butter or romaine) for wrapping

Instructions:

1. In a bowl, combine the chopped hard-boiled eggs, mayonnaise, Dijon mustard, diced celery, chopped fresh dill, salt, and pepper. Mix well.
2. Place a scoop of the egg salad mixture onto each lettuce leaf.
3. Roll up the lettuce leaves, enclosing the egg salad.
4. Secure with toothpicks if needed.
5. Serve the egg salad lettuce wraps as a serotonin-boosting and light meal or snack.

Baked Eggs in Tomato Cups

Ingredients:

- 4 large tomatoes
- 4 eggs
- 1/4 cup grated Parmesan cheese
- 2 tablespoons chopped fresh basil
- Salt and pepper to taste

Instructions:

1. Preheat the oven to 375°F (190°C).
2. Cut off the tops of the tomatoes and scoop out the seeds and pulp, creating a hollow cup.
3. Place the hollowed tomatoes on a baking dish.
4. Crack one egg into each tomato cup, being careful not to overflow.
5. Sprinkle grated Parmesan cheese, chopped fresh basil, salt, and pepper over each egg.
6. Bake in the preheated oven for about 15-20 minutes or until the eggs are cooked to your desired level of doneness.
7. After taking them out of the oven, give them some time to cool.

8. Serve the baked eggs in tomato cups as a serotonin-boosting and visually appealing breakfast or brunch option.

PINEAPPLE

RECIPE FEATURING PINEAPPLE

Pineapple Smoothie

Ingredients:

- 1 cup of chunks of fresh pineapple
- 1 ripe banana
- Coconut milk, or any other non-dairy milk, in a cup
- 1 tablespoon chia seeds
- 1 tablespoon maple syrup or honey (optional, for extra sweetness)
- Ice cubes (optional)

Instructions:

1. In a blender, combine fresh pineapple chunks, ripe banana, coconut milk, chia seeds, honey or maple syrup (if using), and ice cubes (if desired).
2. Blend on high until smooth and creamy.
3. If the smoothie is too thick, you can add more coconut milk or water to reach your desired consistency.

4. Pour into a glass and enjoy the refreshing and serotonin-boosting pineapple smoothie.

Grilled Pineapple Skewers

Ingredients:

- 1 pineapple, peeled and cored
- 2 tablespoons honey
- 1 tablespoon lime juice
- Pinch of cinnamon (optional)
- 30-minute-soaked wooden skewers in water

Instructions:

1. Preheat the grill to medium-high heat.
2. Cut the pineapple into chunks or slices.
3. In a small bowl, mix honey, lime juice, and cinnamon (if using).
4. Thread the pineapple pieces onto the soaked wooden skewers.
5. Brush the pineapple skewers with the honey-lime mixture, coating them evenly.

6. Place the skewers on the grill and cook for about 2-3 minutes per side, until the pineapple has grill marks and is slightly caramelized.
7. After removing off the grill, give them some time to cool.
8. Serve the grilled pineapple skewers as a serotonin-boosting and delightful snack or dessert.

Pineapple Fried Rice

Ingredients:

- 2 cups cooked rice (preferably chilled)
- 1 cup pineapple chunks
- 1/2 cup diced bell peppers (any color)
- 1/2 cup diced carrots
- 1/2 cup peas
- 1/4 cup diced onion
- 2 cloves garlic, minced
- 2 tablespoons soy sauce
- 1 tablespoon vegetable oil
- 1 tablespoon curry powder (optional)
- Salt and pepper to taste
- Chopped cilantro or green onions for garnish

Instructions:

1. In a big skillet or wok, heat the vegetable oil over medium-high heat.
2. To the skillet, add diced onion and garlic. Sauté until aromatic for about a minute.
3. Add diced bell peppers, diced carrots, and peas to the skillet. Cook for a few minutes until the vegetables are crisp-tender.
4. Push the vegetables to one side of the skillet and add chilled cooked rice to the other side.
5. Stir-fry the rice for a couple of minutes to break up any clumps and heat it through.
6. Add soy sauce and curry powder (if using) to the skillet, and mix well with the vegetables and rice.
7. Add pineapple chunks to the skillet and toss everything together.
8. Cook the pineapple for a further minute or two until well cooked.
9. Season with salt and pepper to taste.
10. Remove from heat and garnish with chopped cilantro or green onions.
11. Serve the pineapple fried rice as a serotonin-boosting and flavorful meal.

Pineapple Teriyaki Chicken

Ingredients:

- 2 cubed, skinless, boneless chicken breasts
- 1 cup fresh pineapple chunks
- 1/4 cup low-sodium soy sauce
- 2 tablespoons honey
- 1 tablespoon rice vinegar
- 1 tablespoon cornstarch
- 1 tablespoon vegetable oil
- 2 cloves garlic, minced
- 1 teaspoon grated fresh ginger
- Salt and pepper to taste
- Cooked rice for serving

Instructions:

1. In a small bowl, whisk together soy sauce, honey, rice vinegar, cornstarch, salt, and pepper to make the teriyaki sauce.
2. In a big skillet or wok, heat the vegetable oil over medium-high heat.

3. Add minced garlic and ginger to the skillet. Sauté for about a minute, until fragrant.
4. Cook the chicken cubes in the skillet until they are thoroughly cooked and browned.
5. Add the pineapple chunks to the skillet and cook for a few minutes until they are heated through.
6. Pour the teriyaki sauce over the chicken and pineapple in the skillet. Stir well to coat everything evenly.
7. Cook for another one or two minutes, or until the sauce starts to slightly thicken.
8. Serve the pineapple teriyaki chicken over cooked rice for a serotonin-boosting and delicious meal.

Pineapple Salsa

Ingredients:

- 1 cup fresh pineapple, diced
- 1/2 cup diced red bell pepper
- 1/4 cup diced red onion
- 1 jalapeno pepper, seeded and finely chopped
- Juice of 1 lime
- 2 tablespoons chopped fresh cilantro

- Salt and pepper to taste

Instructions:

1. In a bowl, combine diced pineapple, diced red bell pepper, diced red onion, and chopped jalapeno pepper.
2. Add the lime juice and chopped fresh cilantro to the bowl.
3. Season with salt and pepper to taste.
4. Mix everything together until well combined.
5. Let the pineapple salsa sit for at least 15 minutes to allow the flavors to meld together.
6. Serve the pineapple salsa as a serotonin-boosting and refreshing accompaniment to grilled meats, fish, or as a dip with tortilla chips.

RECIPE FEATURING TOFU

Tofu Stir-Fry

Ingredients:

- drained and cut into cubes one brick of firm tofu
- 2 cups of a variety of veggies, including carrots, snap peas, bell peppers, and broccoli
- 2 cloves garlic, minced
- 2 tablespoons soy sauce
- 1 tablespoon sesame oil
- 1 tablespoon maple syrup or honey
- 1 tablespoon cornstarch
- 2 tablespoons water
- Salt and pepper to taste
- Cooked rice or noodles for serving

Instructions:

1. In a small bowl, whisk together soy sauce, sesame oil, maple syrup or honey, cornstarch, water, salt, and pepper to make the sauce.

2. In a big skillet or wok, heat a tablespoon of oil over medium-high heat.
3. When the garlic is fragrant, add it to the skillet and cook for approximately a minute.
4. Add the tofu cubes to the skillet and cook until browned on all sides.
5. Add the mixed vegetables to the skillet and stir-fry for a few minutes until crisp-tender.
6. Over the tofu and veggies in the skillet, pour the sauce. To evenly coat everything, thoroughly stir.
7. Till the sauce thickens, cook for one or two more minutes.
8. Serve the tofu stir-fry over cooked rice or noodles for a serotonin-boosting and satisfying meal.

Tofu Scramble

Ingredients:

- 1 block firm tofu, drained and crumbled
- 1/2 cup diced bell peppers
- 1/4 cup diced onion
- 1/4 cup nutritional yeast
- 1 tablespoon soy sauce

- 1 teaspoon turmeric
- 1/2 teaspoon garlic powder
- Salt and pepper to taste
- For garnish, use fresh herbs (such parsley or chives).

Instructions:

1. A skillet with a tablespoon of oil heated to medium-high heat.
2. To the skillet, add diced onions and bell peppers. The vegetables should be sautéed for a few minutes until they are tender.
3. Add crumbled tofu to the skillet and stir well to combine with the vegetables.
4. Sprinkle nutritional yeast, soy sauce, turmeric, garlic powder, salt, and pepper over the tofu mixture.
5. Stir everything together until the tofu is evenly coated with the seasonings.
6. Cook for about 5-7 minutes, stirring occasionally, until the tofu is heated through and resembles the texture of scrambled eggs.
7. Adjust the seasoning if needed.
8. Remove from heat and garnish with fresh herbs.
9. Serve the tofu scramble as a serotonin-boosting and protein-packed breakfast or brunch option.

Teriyaki Tofu Bowl

Ingredients:

- 1 block of firm tofu, drained, and cubed
- 2 cups cooked quinoa or rice
- 1 cup steamed broccoli florets
- 1/2 cup shredded carrots
- 2 green onions, sliced
- 2 tablespoons low-sodium soy sauce
- 1 tablespoon honey or maple syrup
- 1 tablespoon rice vinegar
- 1 tablespoon cornstarch
- 1 tablespoon vegetable oil
- Sesame seeds for garnish (optional)

Instructions:

1. In a small bowl, whisk together soy sauce, honey or maple syrup, rice vinegar, cornstarch, and a tablespoon of water to make the teriyaki sauce.
2. Over medium-high heat, heat the vegetable oil in a skillet.

3. Add the tofu cubes to the skillet and cook until browned on all sides.
4. Pour the teriyaki sauce over the tofu in the skillet. Stir well to coat the tofu with the sauce.
5. Cook for another minute or two until the sauce thickens and glazes the tofu.
6. Divide cooked quinoa or rice among serving bowls.
7. Top with teriyaki tofu, steamed broccoli florets, shredded carrots, and sliced green onions.
8. Sprinkle sesame seeds over the bowl if desired.
9. Serve the teriyaki tofu bowl as a serotonin-boosting and wholesome meal.

Tofu and Vegetable Curry

Ingredients:

- 1 block of firm tofu, drained, and cubed
- 1 can coconut milk
- 2 cups mixed vegetables (such as bell peppers, zucchini, cauliflower, and peas)
- 1 onion, diced
- 2 cloves garlic, minced
- 1 tablespoon curry powder

- 1 teaspoon ground turmeric
- 1 teaspoon ground cumin
- Salt and pepper to taste
- Fresh cilantro for garnish
- Cooked rice or naan bread for serving

Instructions:

1. Heat a tablespoon of oil in a large pot or skillet over medium heat.
2. Add diced onion and minced garlic to the pot. The onion should be transparent after a few minutes of sautéing.
3. Add curry powder, ground turmeric, and ground cumin to the pot. Stir well to coat the onion and garlic with the spices.
4. Add mixed vegetables to the pot and cook for a few minutes until they start to soften.
5. Add the coconut milk, then boil the mixture.
6. Gently add the tofu cubes to the pot and stir to combine.
7. Cover the pot and let the curry simmer for about 10-15 minutes, until the vegetables are tender and the flavors are well combined.
8. Season with salt and pepper to taste.

9. Remove from heat and garnish with fresh cilantro.
10. Serve the tofu and vegetable curry over cooked rice
    or with naan bread for a serotonin-boosting and
    flavorful meal.

Tofu and Veggie Skewers

Ingredients:

- 1 block firm tofu, drained and cut into cubes
- 1 cup mixed vegetables (such as bell peppers, cherry tomatoes, zucchini, and red onion), cut into chunks
- 2 tablespoons soy sauce
- 1 tablespoon maple syrup or honey
- 1 tablespoon olive oil
- 1 tablespoon lemon juice
- 1 teaspoon smoked paprika
- Salt and pepper to taste
- 30-minute-soaked wooden skewers in water

Instructions:

1. To create the marinade, combine the soy sauce, honey, maple syrup, olive oil, lemon juice, smoked paprika, salt, and pepper in a small bowl.
2. Alternating between tofu and vegetables, thread the tofu cubes and mixed veggies onto the moistened wooden skewers.
3. Place the skewers in a shallow dish and pour the marinade over them. Make sure they are well coated.
4. Let the skewers marinate for at least 30 minutes to allow the flavors to infuse.
5. Heat the grill or grill pan to a moderately high temperature.
6. Grill the tofu and veggie skewers for about 10-15 minutes, turning occasionally, until the tofu is browned and the vegetables are tender.
7. After removing off the grill, give them some time to cool.
8. Serve the tofu and veggie skewers as a serotonin-boosting and protein-rich dish.

CONCLUSION

Incorporating serotonin-boosting foods into your diet for overall wellness

Incorporating serotonin-boosting foods into your diet is a beneficial way to promote overall wellness. While serotonin itself cannot be directly obtained from food, certain nutrients and dietary habits can support its production and availability in the brain. By prioritizing these foods, you can enhance your mood, improve sleep, reduce stress, and support cognitive function.

Start by focusing on whole foods as the foundation of your diet. Fruits, vegetables, whole grains, lean meats, and healthy fats are a few of these. Numerous vital minerals found in these foods help the synthesis of serotonin and general well-being. Avoid highly processed foods that are often devoid of nutrients and can have negative effects on your mood and energy levels.

Tryptophan is an amino acid that serves as a building block for serotonin. Include tryptophan-rich items in your diet. Turkey, poultry, eggs, dairy products, almonds, seeds, tofu, and legumes are some excellent sources. By consuming these foods, you can ensure a sufficient supply of tryptophan for serotonin synthesis.

Complex carbohydrates play a role in facilitating the absorption of tryptophan in the brain. Choose whole grains instead, such as whole wheat bread, quinoa, brown rice, and oats. Additionally, include fruits and vegetables such as bananas, sweet potatoes, spinach, and broccoli. These foods not only provide complex carbohydrates but also offer a variety of vitamins, minerals, and fiber for overall health.

Omega-3 fatty acids are known for their positive impact on brain health and mood. Include fatty fish like salmon, mackerel, and sardines in your diet. These fish are rich in omega-3s, which may indirectly support serotonin production. If you follow a plant-based diet, incorporate flaxseeds, chia seeds, and walnuts as alternative sources of omega-3 fatty acids.

Vitamin B6 is crucial for the conversion of tryptophan into serotonin. Ensure adequate intake of this vitamin by including foods such as bananas, spinach, avocados, poultry, fish, sunflower seeds, and chickpeas in your diet.

A healthy gut is essential for optimal serotonin production. Include fermented foods like yogurt, kefir, sauerkraut, kimchi, and kombucha in your diet. These foods contain beneficial bacteria that support gut health and may indirectly influence serotonin levels.

To maximize the benefits of serotonin-boosting foods, practice balanced meals that include a combination of protein, complex carbohydrates, and healthy fats. This approach helps regulate blood sugar levels and provides a steady supply of tryptophan for serotonin production.

Finally, it's important to practice mindful eating habits. Pay attention to your body's hunger and fullness cues, and avoid restrictive diets or skipping meals, as they can negatively impact serotonin levels and overall well-being.

The importance of a balanced diet for optimal brain function

A balanced diet is crucial for optimal brain function as it provides the necessary nutrients, energy, and support for the brain's structure, development, and cognitive processes. The brain requires a constant supply of nutrients to function efficiently, and a balanced diet ensures that these nutritional needs are met. Some key reasons why a balanced diet is essential for optimal brain function:

Energy Supply: The brain is a highly energy-demanding organ, accounting for about 20% of the body's total energy expenditure. Glucose, derived from carbohydrates, is the primary source of energy for the brain. Consuming complex carbohydrates, such as whole grains, fruits, and vegetables, provides a steady release of glucose, ensuring a constant energy supply to the brain. This helps maintain focus, concentration, and overall cognitive performance.

Essential Nutrients: A balanced diet provides essential nutrients that are vital for brain health and function. These include vitamins, minerals, antioxidants, and omega-3 fatty acids. For example, B vitamins (found in whole grains, leafy greens, and legumes) support neurotransmitter synthesis and energy metabolism, while antioxidants (found in colorful fruits and vegetables) protect the brain from oxidative stress. Omega-3 fatty acids (found in fatty fish, flaxseeds, and walnuts) are crucial for brain development, neurotransmitter function, and inflammation regulation.

Neurotransmitter Production: Neurotransmitters are chemicals that facilitate communication between brain cells. A balanced diet ensures an adequate supply of amino acids, vitamins, and minerals needed for neurotransmitter synthesis. For example, proteins from sources like lean meats, poultry, fish, legumes, and dairy products provide the amino acids required for neurotransmitter production. Serotonin, dopamine, and norepinephrine are examples of neurotransmitters that influence mood, motivation, and cognitive function.

Brain Growth and Development: Proper nutrition is particularly important for brain growth and development, especially during childhood and adolescence. Nutrients like iron, zinc, iodine, choline, and essential fatty acids play crucial roles in brain development, neuronal connectivity, and cognitive function. Including nutrient-rich foods like lean proteins, whole grains, eggs, nuts, seeds, and leafy greens supports optimal brain growth and function during these critical periods.

Cognitive Performance and Mental Health: A balanced diet directly affects cognitive performance, memory, learning, and overall mental health. Research suggests that deficiencies in specific nutrients, such as omega-3 fatty acids, B vitamins, vitamin D, and magnesium, may impair cognitive function and increase the risk of mental health disorders such as depression, anxiety, and age-related cognitive decline. On the other hand, a diet rich in fruits, vegetables, whole grains, lean proteins, and healthy fats has been associated with better cognitive performance, improved mood, and reduced risk of mental health issues.

FINAL THOUGHTS AND RECOMMENDATIONS

When it comes to incorporating serotonin-boosting foods into your diet, it's important to prioritize a variety of nutrient-dense options. Aim for a diverse and balanced diet that includes a wide range of foods. This ensures that you receive a broad spectrum of nutrients that support serotonin production and overall well-being.

It's also crucial to consider individual needs when incorporating these foods. Factors such as age, sex, activity level, and any underlying health conditions can impact your nutritional requirements. Therefore, it's recommended to consult with a registered dietitian or healthcare professional to receive personalized advice tailored to your specific needs.

While diet plays a role in serotonin production, it's important to adopt a holistic approach to well-being. Factors such as regular physical activity, stress management, quality sleep, and social connections also influence serotonin levels and overall wellness. Therefore, it's essential to pay attention to these aspects of your lifestyle in conjunction with a serotonin-boosting diet.

Practicing mindful eating habits is crucial when incorporating serotonin-boosting foods into your diet. Pay attention to your body's hunger and fullness signs, take your time eating, and slow down. This can help prevent overeating or undereating and promote a balanced approach to nutrition.

Moderation is key when it comes to incorporating serotonin-boosting foods. While these foods can support serotonin production, it's important to maintain a balanced approach and avoid excessive consumption of any particular food or nutrient. Remember to prioritize a variety of foods and maintain a well-rounded diet.

Personalizing your diet is another important aspect to consider. Experiment with different serotonin-boosting foods and recipes to find what works best for you. Incorporate these foods into your favorite dishes or try new recipes to make your meals enjoyable and satisfying.

In some cases, dietary supplements may be recommended to support serotonin levels. However, it's crucial to consult with a healthcare professional before starting any supplements, as they can interact with medications or have potential side effects.